Intermittent Fasting

The Step By Step Guide For Beginners

Effective Path To Optimal Health And Healthy Weight Loss

Wild Goose Media Publications

Amy Fisher

For Those in the "mountains"

(You Know Who You Are)

Table of Contents

Introduction

Pssst! Yes! You over there!

Looks like you are searching for some ways to lose fat and achieve weight loss and you have chanced upon this topic of Intermittent Fasting. First off, I would like to extend a warm welcome and bid you make yourself comfortable as we move in and explore this domain of Intermittent Fasting. I am really glad you are here, as you will be getting loads of value as well as plenty of actionable strategies which will undoubtedly be useful in boosting your weight loss journey to the next level!

I would like to say that I am by no means the primary authoritative figure when it comes to Intermittent Fasting. The main reason why I labored on this book and its useful store of information is just because I felt compelled to share all that I have learnt and experienced about this particular topic. Intermittent fasting made me relook the way I lived and in the process, saved my life.

I was in a bad way prior to my discovery of intermittent fasting. Being an overweight, borderline obese, single mother coping with her new born, whilst grappling with a sizeable host of physical ailments would not be something that I would wish on anyone. Faced with such odds, I did what most folks would do – try to get a quick solution to all the problems and medicate my way out of the mess.

That did not work.

It wasn't until intermittent fasting made its way into my life that I finally managed to address the root cause of my many physical ailments – namely my weight. Things have changed dramatically since then, which is why this book is meant to share all that I have learned as a result of practicing intermittent fasting for more than half a decade and aims to put out everything on the subject in a simple yet comprehensive and understandable manner to help you make the right decisions for yourself.

Intermittent fasting as a topic has been pretty trendy, with loads of celebrities like Hugh Jackman as well as Jennifer Lopez swearing by its weight loss and fat burning results. It isn't just the stars in Tinseltown who seem to have benefited though. Many others who have taken up fasting also see great, sustainable results with regards to their health and weight. Fasting is by no means a fad. In reality, it has been practiced by many since the ancient times as a concurrent means of spiritual and physiological healing.

This book goes into the various topics surrounding intermittent fasting, ranging from the different methods of fasting to the veritable host of benefits that one gets when incorporating intermittent fasting into your lifestyle. Structured with a step by step guide on how to actually prepare for and start a fast, it also delves into how a simple fast can actually snowball into many positives like overall lowered inflammation of the body, improved energy levels as well as the auto triggering of the body's natural fat burning process.

In my humble opinion, the value of this book lies in the fact that it gives a detailed rundown of almost everything that is available on the subject in order to help you develop a thorough understanding of what Intermittent Fasting is and what it entails (or not!). This is coupled fastidiously with the important How-To aspects of implementing a fast so that it is sustainable and long lasting for you to enjoy all the great benefits that intermittent fasting has to offer.

It is not implied, in any way, shape or form, that Intermittent Fasting is the be all and end all magical solution to all of the health issues around the world! Rather it advocates a sensible incorporation of the practice into your lifestyle and then being an avid observer of what it unfolds for you and your loved ones.

In my case, it was mostly great things which is why I present to you this book in the knowledge and hope that Intermittent Fasting does the same for you as it has done for me.

See you around the fasting bandwagon! Please do enjoy the boosted weight loss, better health and improved lifestyle while you are at it!

Finding the best at your worst

Before we take a deep dive into this book, let me add a little note that will hopefully get any erroneous assumptions you might have about the contents of this book out of the way.

If you think that I am going to preach about some brutal gym routine or brag about a popular diet endlessly until it seems only natural, please let me clarify that this won't be the case. Considering the fact that I am a single parent and have been finding it difficult in being able to follow any stringent diet program or exercise routine for more than a week, I can definitely empathize with those of you who are in the same boat as me.

However, despite my not too successful efforts at sticking to an exercise program or any of the low-carb, high-carb whatchamacallit diets out there, I can safely say that I am in a much better place mentally and physically than I have ever been before.

In fact, it won't be an overstatement to say that I never experienced a more healthy state of mind and body in my entire life!

Don't get me wrong though. I am aware that there are folks out there who consistently make time for the gym and would never as much as touch a single piece of food that their diet plan prohibits. I am not implying, under any circumstances, that these individuals are doing anything wrong. Quite the contrary, doing all that and more on a daily, consistent basis would probably require an iron will and steely determination. Something which we ought to commend and applaud them for. However, what about those of us who aren't that well-endowed with an unwavering resolve and an ironclad self-control? Does it mean that our quest for better health and sustainable weight loss would be doomed to failure?

I should think not!

After all, I would be the first to admit that I was never a real fan of super strict, restrictive diets and crazily strenuous exercise routines.

Which is why I request you not to doubt my sanity when I say that being healthy is completely possible without restricting yourself to a meticulous diet and exercise plan.

How did I do it? The same way that you would be doing, once you get started on the Intermittent Fasting lifestyle.

Intermittent fasting transformed me from a miserable new mom suffering from various health issues (including the worst postpartum depression and anxiety) to someone who is utterly confident in herself and her health. Having found myself in the best shape possible (physically, mentally and emotionally) has allowed me to secure a well-paying full time job, enjoy raising the most beautiful, self-assured and happy little boy and revel in life like never before!

And in all honesty, those are just some (albeit the biggest) perks I have been able to enjoy because of practicing intermittent fasting.

Now, you might be wondering how in the world did I encounter this awesome lifestyle change in the first place.

The reality is, I discovered Intermittent Fasting when I wasn't even looking for it!

And while the above statement in itself might make it seem like it is less of a practice or imply that it is something that I take for granted - that isn't true in the slightest.

In fact, I will go as far as to admit that once I discovered intermittent fasting, my life changed completely and I was introduced to another level of health and well-being that I had never experienced before.

Sounds intriguing, right?

The results that I obtained within merely a year of fasting intermittently were remarkable enough. However, the benefits I have experienced over the span of more than five years of practicing intermittent fasting is what compelled me to share this truly magical regimen that transformed my life.

I understand that our health problems and life dilemmas may differ, but my story aims to inspire you to understand how something as simple as intermittent fasting transformed so many areas of my life. All at once.

And how it has the potential to change yours too!

What follows is a brief account of how I actually discovered intermittent fasting. Apart from anything else, I hope that it gives you some hope in life and the courage to deal with the adversities you might be facing.

I first encountered intermittent fasting when I was at the lowest point of my life and least expecting a health revolution. I was a sad and overweight single parent in her mid 30s, struggling with a multitude of health problems (and a fussy baby) and felt the loneliest I have ever been in my life because my baby's daddy had just left me.

I was also grappling with the worst form of postpartum depression and was consequently highly emotionally vulnerable. On top of all that, I had developed hypertension during pregnancy which didn't quite improve even after delivery and was diagnosed with hypothyroidism soon after giving birth. Trying to get the hang of dealing with the needs of a newborn while managing my own health issues and juggling the unending demands of being an only parent made up some of the most challenging times of my life.

I wasn't coping well and got extremely exhausted by my miserable existence after a few months, and the whole situation seemed particularly devastating when I looked at my baby's innocent face and realized that my poor health was having a direct impact on my little angel.

But I was yet to be hit hard by the severity of our plight.

Nothing made the austerity of my health problems more evident than an incident that had me witness first-hand how my deteriorating physical and mental health was taking a serious toll on my child.

It was like an eye-opener for me that shook my whole being.

And in the aftermath, I found myself changed forever.

My maternity leave had just ended and it was my first week back at work. As if returning to the office after a harrowing experience with childbirth and looking after a newborn wasn't already enough, I found my depression and anxiety go through the roof. Each morning as I left for work, I found myself sobbing as both my baby and I felt the worst separation anxiety there is to experience.

However, life had to go on and I could not afford to take an unpaid leave at the moment which is why I gathered myself together as best as I could and tried to focus on my work in an attempt to divert my mind. But while I might have been somewhat successful at coping with the situation, my baby was still struggling with it.

And struggling badly, for that matter.

And the worst part was that I had no idea about my poor child's struggles.

One day while I was at work, my mom called hysterically and informed in a panic-stricken voice that Jason (my baby boy) won't stop crying and that she thought he couldn't breathe because of it. My mom was so horrified looking at Jason's face (which was turning bluer with each passing moment!) that she didn't even call an ambulance but rang me instead and shouted at the top of her lungs for me to return this very second.

I rushed towards home as soon as she hung up and called an ambulance on my way back. Long story short, the doctors in the emergency room diagnosed Jason with a pretty bad panic attack. They had to give him oxygen to improve his breathing and were finally able to calm him down after 30 minutes of continuous efforts.

As the doctors briefed me about his situation 45 minutes later, all I could see were blurred faces and hear their muffled voices. The only thing that stuck with me was this; my four-month old child just had a panic attack!

Further investigations into the matter revealed that my uncontrollable anxiety was somehow acquired by Jason. The psychologist explained to me that a stressed parent is more likely to be distant, less engaged and incompatible in meeting their child's physical and emotional needs no matter how hard they think they're trying. Moreover, he also told me that babies can actually feel the disturbing emotions of their parents, such as fear and sadness, and can be directly affected by them.

I was also informed that I needed to work on my own mental and physical well-being if I wanted my baby to be healthy and happy.

And not have an even more severe panic attack next time around.

Who would have known that my health was affecting my child so profoundly and that my own well-being was linked that strongly to that of my kid's?

The reality hit me, and it hit me hard!

Neglecting my own mental and physical health was like disregarding my baby's. And I never wanted any of that.

Which is why I promised myself that very day that I will be striving hard to become a healthy individual, mentally and physically, and be the best version of myself for my child's sake. And it wasn't just some self-affirmatory mantra or feel good hype when I made that resolution. Deep down, I knew that the years of neglecting my health had finally caught up with me, and now my child and I had to face the music.

The months that ensued were filled with relentless research and talking to various doctors, nutritionists and diet experts in order to find a healthy and sustainable lifestyle that would suit me as a 24/7-on-call single parent.

I literally gave most of the diets a serious go (I kid you not), because I really wanted to get myself out of this worsening health spiral. But each honest attempt at following those restrictive diets came to naught and I seriously was at a loss. It wasn't until one of my friends mentioned the concept of intermittent fasting casually when she visited that perked my ears and made me sit up a little straighter.

No dire, restrictive diet and no need for the couple of hours of gym workout? Lose weight and have it stay off? Normalize cholesterol and blood sugar levels? You bet I was very interested when I heard all that from my friend. And I was sucked into an exhaustive search on virtually whatever there was to find on intermittent fasting on and offline. This led me to be able to build a structured, step by step intermittent fasting program that stayed the course and ensure its sustainability in the long run.

And all of this led me to change my life for the better, to say the least.

With the help of intermittent fasting, I transformed myself from an overweight miserable parent to someone who has never been more proud of themselves and how well they're doing in life and as a parent.

Even though I have been practicing Intermittent Fasting for almost half a decade, I started experiencing its tremendous benefits when I was less than a year into consistent practice. For starters, I found myself shedding almost 40 pounds in less than 6 months. Hypertension became a thing of the past while my cholesterol levels finally stopped trying to be so unruly. Quite surprisingly, I also found that I had fewer to zero urges to consume unhealthy food or binge-snack myself to a food coma. And contrary to what you may think, I was more alert and focused during fasting than I normally would be and witnessed my productivity spike during the fasting window.

All within the span of a year.

Progressively, I have found myself in the right headspace to thrive both personally and professionally and have never felt more satisfied and happy with my life.

But the best part is that Jason has grown to be a happy, confident and amazing kid.

Which is the biggest thing this lifestyle change of fasting intermittently has allowed me to achieve.

But I'll admit this much. It is not quite easy to be able to believe in something unless you can be sure that it has some legitimacy to it and know exactly how and why it works. Which is why this book aims to answer all your queries regarding

Intermittent Fasting and help you decide whether the practice is meant for you or not.

Good luck!

Ch 1: What Is All This Fuss?

Is the modern diet killing us?

What we eat can make or break us. However, our diets have altered for the worst in the last few decades. This chapter explains EXACTLY what it is in our diets that is killing us!

Its been a long day and Sara was extremely exhausted. A quick glance at the clock made her realize that almost 10 hours had passed since she last ate. As if waiting for that exact moment, her empty stomach growled, confirming her suspicions.

Sara was famished after a tiring day at work and too exhausted to fix a meal for herself. Hearing her stomach begging for food again, she picked up the phone and punched in the number of the nearest burger joint.

Ten minutes later, she was digging into her scrumptious grub and thanking God for the existence of fast food.

Now let's rewind back to a few million years and see what Asher Rosinger and his tribe, including his three wives and thirteen children, are dining on. Asher and his tribe are hunter-gatherers and roam about in search of anything they can consume. A wild pig or antelope usually forebodes a good hunting day but a giant bison or a couple of gigantic mammoths would mean a feast for everyone.

Tonight their menu includes some mouth-watering boar, a generous serving of scrumptious tubers as well as fresh mangoes and grapefruit plucked directly from the trees.

Can you recognize how dramatically our diets have changed over the decades?

Granted, we have come a long way from the stone age in terms of the time that has passed and the technology that has evolved, but so have our diets. As humans mastered agriculture and commercial farming made some remarkable progress, this change was inevitable AND necessary for survival, to say the least. However, the important question to ask is whether this agricultural revolution and transformation has turned out in our favor?

The answer is not quite straightforward and one has to dig a little deeper to find out why the modern diet may not be the blessing we consider it to be.

Are you ready?

Let me begin by saying this:

Modern food is the leading cause of mortality worldwide...

But before you take me as the world's worst critic, let me explain.

I understand that the image of Sara digging into her appetizing burger and flavoursome fries makes the above statement hard to believe. Add in the garlic mayo dip she is enjoying, the chicken nuggets that were sent as a free add-on and the cold and refreshing fizzy drink that she sips on every now and then, and one would want to ignore this fact altogether.

But, can we?

Can we disregard the fact that we might be eating and drinking ourselves to death?

Is the modern diet slowly killing us?

These are some critical and probing questions that might tease an inquisitive mind. Therefore, let's look into all the twisted reasons the modern diet is a bigger exterminator of the human race than alcohol or tobacco.

Yeah, you read that last part right.

What we don't know about our food!

The Division for Heart Disease and Stroke Prevention of the CDC (Centers for Disease Control and Prevention) reports that 1 in every 3 adults in America suffers from high blood pressure. It also goes on to state that 1 in every 3 American adults has prehypertension, which implies that their blood pressure is higher than normal but not yet in the hypertension range.

High blood pressure raises the risk for heart diseases and stroke, which are the two leading causes of death in America. It led or contributed to more than 472,000 deaths in 2017.

That amounts to approximately 1300 people breathing their last each day!

But that's not all. According to the National Diabetes Statistics Report (2017) of the CDC, a total of 30.3 million people in the U.S (or 9.4% of the population) have diabetes. In addition to those who actually have it, 33.9% of the adult population in the country has prediabetes, implying that they are extremely close to being diagnosed with type 2 diabetes.

Diabetes is the 7th leading cause of death in the U.S and, according to the CDC, causes 79,535 deaths per year. The American Diabetes Association (ADA) goes as far as to state that Diabetes kills more people annually than AIDS and breast cancer combined.

But wait. There's more!?

The CDC also reports that 33% of the U.S population suffers from high cholesterol, which is a critical risk factor for heart diseases.

And the fact that these heart diseases claim the highest number of lives in the country reinforces the gravity of this health dilemma.

One look at these grim statistics on High Blood Pressure, Diabetes and Elevated Cholesterol levels, and the mind feels obligated to figure out why our overall health has been deteriorating over the years.

Here's why.

A *MAJOR* factor that contributes to all the diseases mentioned above, and many more, is our diet.

Yes. What we consume each and every day has more far reaching effects on our health than we care to acknowledge.

But why is something that is meant for our sustenance be killing us?

Maybe the reasons outlined below will explain.

A spike in sugar intake

Our obsession with sugar dates as far back as millions of years ago when our ancestors (the apes) relied on the consumption of sugary foods such as fruit to gain energy and help store fat for winters. That was a good strategy back then. The hunter-gatherer lifestyle as well as the uncertainty and limited nature of food supplies these early humans relied upon made the consumption of any sugars, carbs and proteins these folks could get their hands on a critical factor for survival.

Not so much for the modern homo sapien though.

We do not live within the same conditions that our ancestors had to survive in. Most of us have plenty of food all year round, including off season fruits and veggies that were only once available during a specific season. While this may sound like a great achievement, particularly when compared to the archaic agricultural and farming practices our ancestral counterparts had to rely on, it has come with a price.

In addition to consuming produce that has been genetically modified to look, taste and feel good, modern food is chock-full of processed sugars (we are age-old buddies with sugar, remember?). Combined with the increased consumption of soda (aka sugar bomb) and fruit juice, our bodies are exposed to a sugar surge they aren't programmed to handle.

The results, not quite surprisingly, present themselves in the form of insulin resistance and diabetes.

High consumption of (mostly empty) calories

While consuming calories is critical to the proper functioning of our bodies, the key is to consume the right amount through optimum sources that provide not just any calories but nutrient-rich calories.

In this context, the problem with modern diet is that it is brimming with processed foods that provide empty calories but no nutrition. While this means that a person consuming a burger may feel full and satisfied, they haven't eaten anything that could be of nutritional value to their body. As our brain detects a lack of nutrition coming from the appetizing meal one is busy chomping down, it keeps signalling the body to crave for more food in hopes that some nutrition can be obtained.

Modern food has also been engineered to please our taste buds and the reward systems in our brain so one just cannot stop munching on them and gain excess weight without getting any nutrition whatsoever.

The consequences range from obesity and heart disease to diabetes and depression.

Healthy fats replaced with, well... some really unhealthy ones

There was a time when people consumed butter, lard and other healthy fats and were relatively leaner individuals with lesser heart problems and lived happily ever after.

But what went wrong? And when?

It all started with the misconception that all fats were created equal and were bad for us, leading to obesity and heart disease. The idea particularly went viral after World War II when many studies endorsed the connection between heart disease and saturated fats. What followed on was a widespread withdrawal from traditional healthy fats such as butter, lard, and coconut oil in favor of highly processed vegetable oils including sunflower, corn and canola oils in an attempt to reduce weight and have a healthier heart.

So much for healthy food choices, huh?

These new and advanced varieties of oils contain a high proportion of Omega-6 fatty acids which can cause inflammation as well as invite a host of other dysfunctions in the body when consumed in excess. Additionally, the fact that these oils could quickly go rancid owing to the highly sensitive polyunsaturated fats found in them gave way to another dilemma. The solution was found in solidifying them through hydrogenation, which makes them high in trans fats, some of the worst forms of fats for human health.

What's more, while the consumption of traditional fats satiated hunger through smaller meals and kept one full for longer periods, these modern oils manufactured with advanced technologies make it challenging to avoid consuming a higher number of calories. Resultantly, we are exactly how we did not want to be; obese, overweight individuals with high levels of (the very harmful) LDL cholesterol and inflammation, and more heart issues than ever before.

Processed foods taking over our lives

Can you recall the number of times you've simply popped open a packet of microwave ramen noodles and enjoyed your favorite snack-time meal within a span of five to seven minutes, tops?

Or how often, in the midst of all that morning madness, you've decided that a bowl of cereal would suffice as breakfast?

From the canned veggies you use in your salads to that hot pizza that is promised to be delivered under 20 minutes, processed foods have more or less taken over our lives. The consumption of fast food has dramatically increased in the past few decades and an ever increasing number of people are consuming pre-packaged 'convenience' foods that are detrimental to human health.

These processed foods contain harmful chemicals in the form of artificial flavors and preservatives as well as inflammatory vegetable oils and a huge amount of non-nutritious calories. Additionally, they are overloaded with salts, sugar, and high fructose corn syrup that act as taste enhancers and make us crave these foods.

Even when all they do is destroy our health.

In short, processed foods have practically ambushed our lives and are slowly but surely killing us.

And you thought that microwave ramen was H.E.A.V.E.N.L.Y.

The evolution of farming practices-much to our detriment

The paleolithic societies that existed in the stone age depended primarily on hunting, fishing and foraging. These hunter-gatherers lived together in small groups and pretty much lived like nomads.

But there were some major problems with this vagabond lifestyle...

Not only did these early humans have to forage for food, fight for it with all they had if it came to that, and migrate from a place when the food resources in that area were depleted, they also had yet to find a way to make these food crops depend on them instead of the other way round.

But that had to change if the survival of the human race was to be ensured. And it did.

Approximately 12,000 years ago, humans began farming and started playing with the idea of domesticating animals. This marked the beginning of the Neolithic Revolution (also known as the 'Agricultural Revolution') and was a time when our ancestral counterparts preserved seeds from the best crops and crossbred different varieties in search of bigger and better produce. Several thousand years later, researchers from the Grantham Centre for Sustainable Futures at the University of Sheffield found that this domestication of crops also increased the seed size of certain vegetables without any deliberate effort on part of the farmers.

We were making some progress as the human race. Great!

But that was just the beginning. Fast forward to the 20th century and we humans were living in an era which was marked by the use of advanced machinery, chemical fertilizers and deadly pesticides and herbicides.

Then came the GMO crops that were genetically modified with built-in pesticides and insecticides. These were artificially engineered to increase crop yield, reduce the costs of food production, enhance nutrient composition and food quality as well as provide medical benefits to the ever increasing world population.

So far so good.

But while all of this was primarily done in an attempt to sustain the ever increasing population of the human race on this planet, these biocides and GMO plants paradoxically introduced some deadly toxins into our systems as we consumed them as well as the milk and meat of animals that were raised on them. In his book 'The Plant Paradox', Dr. Steven R. Gundry explains that these malicious chemicals enter our bodies through the intestinal tract or via skin, thereby messing up with our body genetic programs and leading to various dysfunctions in our bodies.

What even worsens this whole scenario is that the land on which these crops are farmed no longer comprises of the same nutrient-dense rich soil due to mono cropping (farming the same crops on the same piece of land each year). This means that the wheat we consume today isn't as nutritious as it was a good few hundred years ago. This also implies that farmers are now under additional pressure to use chemical fertilizers to enhance the performance of their farmland and crops.

Which might increase production volume and quality, but isn't as good for our health as consuming the produce back then.

The dilemma with our livestock

As we discussed in the previous section, the herbicides and insecticides used in commercial farming get into our system when we consume the milk and meat from animals raised on the said crops. Approximately 100% of the animals raised industrially in farms are fed on GMO crops. The altered genes from these crops not only contaminate the milk, meat and fat of these animals but can also be traced in our systems as we consume these animal products.

But there is more to this dilemma...

Just as plant crops are genetically modified to be more weather resistant or produce their own insecticides, animals are also widely engineered with, for example, growth hormones to reduce the time it takes for them to become ready for the consumer market.

These farm raised animals are also fed with antibiotics to help protect them from an onslaught of diseases that prevail naturally in the extremely unhygienic and cramped-up spaces they are raised and transported in. Additionally, instead of grazing in pastures like they traditionally used to, these animals are fed on highly inflammatory diets of corn, soy and grains that they were never designed to eat or digest.

Upon consumption, the antibiotics that these animals have been administered as well as the harmful substances from the corn and soy they eat transfer into our bodies and wreak havoc on our bodily systems.

As Dr. Steven R. Gundry very matter-of-factly points out:

You are what you eat and what you ate, eat.

Another critical problem with the modern diet, besides the diet itself, is our eating habits and lifestyles. Not only is the modern-day life characterised by a sedentary way of living, but it is also marked with crazy food trends that are sometimes downright astonishing (think charcoal lattes and dessert hummus!). The modern human has an ever growing plethora of food options available to them with just a single tap on their smartphones. This has made giving in to our food cravings ever more easy and enticing.

Ironically, while many of us might be faithful followers of a contemporary diet such as 'Paleo' or 'Keto', our ancestors ate whatever they could get their hands on depending on their geography, season, opportunity, and obviously, fate. This lends immense credit to the belief that humans were evolved to eat the most varied diet possible and that narrowing our focus on certain foods may actually be depriving us of some much needed nutritional value.

Among all this craziness going around in our lives with fad diets, weird eating patterns and toxic food, it becomes even more crucial to be mindful of what we put into our bodies and when.

Which brings us back to the topic of this book.

However, everything has a history (except those weird food combos trending on Snapchat). Care to find out where Intermittent Fasting originated from?

Then please turn the page and on to the next chapter!

Ch 2: The Real Facts And Why You Need To Know

Does history and science lend support to the hype?

Is Intermittent Fasting backed by history and science? Can we jump into this regimen satisfied that it isn't some hippie tradition that is meant to soothe the egos of the nonconformists? Read on to find some answers to questions like these. And much more!

Fasting came naturally to our species, but without us being consciously aware of it at first.

Humans didn't always practice fasting intentionally, which was prehistorically just an unintended consequence of scarce food that these early fellas had to rely on. While many historians believe that we underestimate the resourcefulness of the paleolithic humans and their ability to forage food for themselves, it is nonetheless a reality that the life of the prehistoric human was characterised by good and bad food days.

And in between these feast and famine cycles, they had virtually no choice but to fast.

Neat.

However, as human beings evolved, they learned more about fasting and its virtues and thereby began practicing it consciously. To give you a better understanding of what the modern human deems fasting to be, let's have a look at the definition below.

Encyclopaedia Britannica defines fasting as:

> '...abstinence from food or drink or both for health, ritualistic, religious, or ethical purposes. The abstention may be complete or partial, lengthy, of short duration, or intermittent.'

The Encyclopaedia also goes on to construe fasting as an antique practice stating that it has been historically pursued by physicians, religious founders and common individuals alike. In this context, fasting has proven to be quite a diverse mechanism. The Ancient Greek physician 'Hippocrates' (aka the father of medicine) used to recommend fasting to his patients who exhibited certain symptoms. He is reported to have said,

"To eat when you are sick, is to feed your illness"

-Hippocrates

The Ancient Greeks were such strong proponents of fasting for medicinal purposes that they called it 'the physician within'. They believed that fasting was a remedy ingrained in nature which is why any sick human or animal won't eat properly or stop eating altogether.

In addition to being utilised as a natural cure for certain ailments, fasting is also considered a means of spiritual warfare in certain religions such as Christianity and Islam. While the Christians believe fasting and praying to be two of the strongest weapons against evil, the Muslims observe fasts throughout the Holy month of Ramadan during which they try to abstain from all kinds of wrongdoings and strive to be a better person.

But that's still not all. Fasting has also been extensively used as an instrument for fulfilling the political and social aspirations of the human race. In 1932, Mahatma Gandhi began a hunger strike to protest against the British Government in a bid to further the Indian independence movement from British colonial rule. Gandhi is reported to have observed a total of 17 fasts during India's freedom movement and is known for having a knack for the practice.

Being something that has been used to a variety of ends, it is quite understandable that fasting has many varieties. Depending on what a person's intentions for the practice are, fasting can vary from a complete abstinence of food and water to sustaining one's needs using only liquids.

Additionally, the time limit for fasting can range anywhere from a few hours in a day to dawn-till-dusk or from a full 24 hours to a few days. There are people who fast periodically as a physical or spiritual cleanse and others who have devoted certain days of a week to abstinence. Still others keep daily fasts for a full month or indulge in fasting every now and then for a few days straight.

In this context, fasting is a rather subjective practice unless factors such as religion, social or cultural obligations make it compulsory. One can fast to wean off a food coma after Thanksgiving or simply take a short break from dining to gear up their mental performance. Additionally, a person can also deny themselves in an attempt to shed off a few extra pounds that have been making them self-conscious or may just want to simplify their eating routine.

However, not all forms of fasting are created equal and allow you to be so flexible.

Which brings us to what we've set out to talk about in this book.

IF-The flexible fast

At the outset, the most important thing to understand about Intermittent Fasting is that it is ***not*** a diet plan. It doesn't tell you *what* to eat rather it aims to regulate when you eat.

And if you are anything like me, that simple fact makes the practice more alluring than anything else. In fact, I think it is one of the main reasons why Intermittent Fasting worked so well for me. I felt liberated from the daunting task of counting calories every time I set out to prepare a meal for myself and it made restaurant guesswork a thing of the past. Additionally, I was eating all the healthy food I loved (including carbs, proteins, fats and what not) and losing weight at the same time.

But things weren't always this easy.

In all honesty, I wouldn't call myself a very disciplined person to begin with. Even after practicing Intermittent Fasting for more than five years and writing this book for you (a task that calls for another level of orderliness), I'll admit that there are days when I have to struggle to be consistent. On top of that, I must say I am not the most hardworking person by nature (Aren't we all? No? Okayy).

With that being said, I do not imply that Intermittent Fasting is made for the faint of will exclusively. However, what I am trying to establish here is the fact that the ease with which this practice can be adopted by anyone is remarkable and that it does make room for those of us who find themselves struggling with their sluggish side.

Now that that's out of the way, let's look into what Intermittent Fasting really is.

Intermittent Fasting (I'll use IF for short) is a popular practice that involves cycling between periods of eating and fasting. As is suggested by some studies, IF cannot only cause a person to lose calories and delay the effects of aging but also improves overall health by combating inflammation and enhancing cardiovascular fitness. It can help a person gain more muscle mass, become leaner and increase their explosive strength (aka the ability to exhibit an advanced level of strength within a short time period). In fact, IF is notoriously used by people who want to lose weight without starving themselves.

But these health benefits are not the only reasons IF has become all trendy. One has to factor in the flexibility offered by this practice to understand why IF was the most highly followed diet in the U.S in 2018, with even Paleo and Gluten-free diets failing to make it to the top position. This popularity continued in 2019, with some folks calling it the defining diet of that year.

Not without a reason though.

Imagine being able to eat whatever you fancy (albeit healthy foods, I cannot focus on this point enough and suggest that you don't take healthy eating lightly at all!) without having to follow a strict diet plan that will leave you longing for that perfect steak or chickpea stew. The only thing you had to do was incorporate a fasting schedule in your routine and restrict eating to a narrow window of time that you've set for yourself.

Sounds like it won't be that difficult. Doesn't it?

Nonetheless, I would still reiterate that you cannot gain any benefit from IF if you take it as an excuse to fast and then binge eat during the designated eating period (more on this later!).

Now that you know some basics about IF, I assume that you must be eager to learn everything there is to know about the practice. However, before we delve deeper into IF, let's discuss if science backs up the stir this latest trend has made in the recent years and stands by the authenticity and effectiveness of this practice.

After all, an inquisitive mind like yours must be wondering why one should be ditching the eating patterns they have followed for as long as they can remember, without a valid reason.

If you ask me, it is even more important to understand the whys and hows behind something in an era when fad diets have become a reality and people indulge in all kinds of crazy and insane stuff no level headed person would even consider doing.

So, brace yourselves for some geeky stuff and let's try to understand the biology that goes on within our bodies.

Does science lend support to the hype?

Side note: I understand that not everyone (including myself) has the patience to plough through all those highly sophisticated scientific concepts. Keeping that in mind, I have tried to explain everything in an easily digestible manner and aim at clarifying things for everyone.

With that out of the way, a short answer to the question in the title is 'pretty much yes'. For the detailed version, please refer below.

The human body has been designed to work in an intricate yet elegant (and sometimes mysterious) way. The workings that sustain us are beautifully interlaced and executed with such perfection that one cannot help but be awed by them.

A similar process is set in motion when we consume food.

But before we delve into some details of this indispensable string of events and try to understand how the food we eat is actually used by our bodies, let me give you a little perspective on the whole thing.

The food we eat is not only a cure for those annoying hunger pangs (or cravings) but is also a source of nourishment and energy our body needs to grow and sustain itself. However, the carbohydrates, proteins and fats we consume in the form of food cannot be directly used by our bodies to provide energy and sustain vital bodily functions. Therefore once consumed, these pass through our digestive tract into the intestines where they are broken down into their constituents glucose (sugar), amino acids and fatty acids respectively. These basic units that constitute the complex substances we have eaten can now be used to provide our bodies with the energy that we use to walk, talk, think and perform other daily functions that are necessary to survive and thrive.

Now, let's see what actually happens when we devour a plateful of, say, garlic butter shrimp pasta (just because I feel like having some now, do you?)

When we eat something, our insulin levels rise. For those of you who aren't aware, insulin is a hormone released by the pancreas that helps our body utilize glucose (sugar) from carbohydrates found in the food we consume. It does so by enabling cells to allow glucose to enter them which then provides the fuel that will help these cells perform their respective functions.

However, sometimes (correction: oftentimes) in this era of junk food and binge eating, we consume more carbs than we can ever use. This means there is additional glucose lying around that exceeds our requirements.

Lo and behold! Here comes the infamous 'insulin' to the rescue again and directs our fat cells to store this excess glucose in the form of fat for later use.

Unfortunately, that later rarely comes and our fat storage builds on.

And on.

And on.

Pausing for a few seconds here, let me explain the process of 'Ketosis' before we continue.

Ketosis is a process that kicks in once our body starts to lack its basic fuel source 'Glucose aka sugar'. In the presence of carbs (and their constituents glucose) there is not much need to burn fat. In fact, there is practically no reason to burn fat in the presence of glucose.

This is because of a number of reasons.

First and foremost, our bodies can store up to 98% of the fat we consume whereas the storage capacity for glucose is much less, prompting our system to use any and all of the available glucose on a priority basis. Secondly, it is light on our metabolic system to burn carbs immediately, instead of first processing them into fat for storage and then converting that fat back to carbs when the need actually arises. And finally, carbs are an approved powerhouse because unlike fat, they can be utilized by all our cells for meeting their energy needs.

To bring home this point, let's think of our brain for a second. Our brain is a vital organ that needs to generate electrical impulses for the neurons (brain cells) to communicate with each other and send vital signals throughout the body that could mean life or death for us. All of that sure sounds impressive, however, the brain needs massive amounts of energy to perform these tasks. So much so that it is regarded as the most energy-consuming organ within the human body.

The only problem with this is that although the brain can use fat for energy, it isn't a very efficient source for fulfilling the organ's tremendous demands since the fat needs to be broken into ketones before it can be used. Furthermore, our brains do not utilize ketones as well as glucose.

Now, do you remember that the excess glucose from the carbs in that shrimp pasta was instructed by insulin to be stored as fat? (No? Maybe you're in a food coma! Just kidding!).

That fat won't be used as long as there is enough glucose in your body because the body's natural mechanism does not allow ketosis to kick in unless there is a chance that the organs will be starved of energy.

However, when we fast, we limit our food intake. For starters, this lowers our insulin levels since the insulin floodgates are opened wide right before and during we eat. Yeah, I still remember. Insulin is good for us, but not too much of it. Excess of anything is bad, even insulin. And too much insulin in our system means we are at a high risk of developing insulin resistance that can lead to prediabetes or type 2 diabetes. Therefore, IF is good in that it suppresses that surge of insulin we get when consuming food thereby preventing our bodies from getting all insulin resistant.

Secondly, IF also creates an opportunity for our bodies to switch to a ketosis mode since there is not enough glucose in the system to generate the energy our cells need to perform their respective functions. Once our fats start burning and provide that alternative (but clean) source of fuel to our bodies, we can see visible results in the form of weight loss.

Therefore, IF is a proven method for losing weight and brings all the health benefits that come with it such as improved cardiovascular health and keeping insulin resistance at bay.

You might be wondering that I haven't talked about proteins and how our bodies use them. Well, proteins are the building blocks of our muscles and, when broken into their constituent units amino acids, build and repair tissues as well as make enzymes, hormones and other body chemicals. They have limited to no contribution when it comes to providing the cells with energy and meet as low as only about 5% of the body's energy needs. Additionally, proteins are left intact until about the third day of fasting when our body has no choice but to break these down for fuel.

This leads us to another science-backed benefit of IF for our physical health. While it triggers the process of ketosis that helps burn away the fat stored in our cells, it also aids in maintaining muscle mass at the same time. This is owing to the fact that although IF deprives us of food for long enough to set off ketosis, it doesn't starve us to the point where our muscles would begin degenerating to provide the much-needed energy.

No wonder people practicing IF experience weight loss while their muscle mass remains intact.

However, your muscle mass isn't only salvaged because proteins are used as a last resort when it comes to providing fuel for the body's normal functionality. It is also spared because fasting brings about some beneficial hormonal changes such as an upsurge in growth hormones and Norepinephrine.

Let's talk about the growth hormones first. Not only does fasting trigger a decrease in the levels of the hormone insulin in the body, it also helps increase the Human Growth Hormone (HGH) which is a counterregulatory hormone whose levels naturally decline as we age. For the purpose of understanding, counterregulatory hormones are the hormones that work against the normal function of insulin; which is to allow the body to either use glucose or store it in the form of fat. A decrease in HGH triggers fat storage as well as causes loss of lean muscle mass, something that is inevitable as the years pass by.

However, fasting induces the release of HGH in adults that results in spiking the blood-glucose levels. This is highly beneficial for us when our body is in the state of fasting and we aren't consuming much carbs or sugar. Additionally, for those of you concerned with a loss of muscle mass during fasting, there is absolutely nothing to worry about. Studies show that the HGH unleashed during fasting likely helps in the maintenance of lean mass – both muscle and bone. There are other studies conducted that also prove that IF is 4 times better at preserving lean mass than calorie-restricted diets.

Amazing, isn't it?

But there's more!

You might remember that in the beginning of this section, I told you how our bodies work in elegant ways. The process I am about to describe will only reinforce this fact.

Studies have found that IF brings about an increase in 'Norepinephrine' levels. Now don't get all baffled by 'Norepinephrine' since it is just a stress hormone that is released during stressful conditions, such as the unavailability of food during fasting.

But how is unleashing a stress hormone in our system beneficial when we've already stretched ourselves thin with fasting?

When we refrain ourselves from eating, the stress hormone Norepinephrine is released so our bodies can be equipped for going out there and forage for food. Just like an armed soldier goes into the battlefield with his gear ready, our bodies are now fully prepared to go out in the world and find grub. The heart rate spikes and blood flow to the muscles increases. There is increased alertness and arousal with a laser sharp focus that aims to help us fulfil the mission of feeding ourselves. And while our nerves are all worked up for the impending call of duty, our bodies rigorously burn fat for fuel so that the engine keeps going. Metabolic activity is raised as high as 3.6%. Now you're ready to take on the world!

And all of this is brought in motion when Norepinephrine is released during the state of fasting.

Our bodies DO work in elegant ways.

Extensive research on the health benefits of IF also shows that there are some other health-related benefits of the practice as well. In a review article published in The New England Journal of Medicine, Mark Mattson (Ph.D) along with Rafael de Cabo (Ph.D), has included some interesting findings about the health benefits of IF.

Mr. Mattson is a John Hopkins University School of Medicine neuroscience professor and former chief of the Laboratory of Neurosciences at the National Institute on Aging. He has been studying IF for almost 25 years while practicing it himself for about 20 years. His article in the NEJM not only confirms the ability of IF to induce 'Metabolic switching', which is essentially the utilization of fats instead of glucose for energy, but also goes on to state a long list of other health benefits of IF. Although the research Mr. Mattson has conducted is primarily on mice and other non-human primates, it is believed that the results could be extended to be applicable to humans.

In his article, Mr. Mattson states that the health benefits of IF are not restricted to weight loss or reduced production of damaging oxygen free radicals, rather IF evokes evolutionary mechanisms in our bodies that improve glucose regulation, increase stress resistance and decrease inflammation. It activates some innate defenses we have against oxidative and metabolic stress and stimulate pathways that remove or repair damaged molecules. For those who don't know what oxidative stress is, it is an imbalance between free radicals and antioxidants in our bodies. While both free radicals and antioxidants are naturally produced by our bodies, their quantities need to be maintained in an intricate balance. An increased amount of free radicals without enough antioxidants to neutralize them can damage cells, proteins and DNA.

Another major benefit of IF that Mr. Mattson explains in his article is increased stress resistance of cells (yeah, our cells get stressed too!). When a person fasts, their cells become stressed (not good). However, when the cells are stressed, they adapt by enhancing their capability to cope with stress (quite good). While doing so, these cells also increase their resistance to disease since they are now in a better shape to deal with all adversities. In this context, Mr. Mattson compares IF to exercise. When we exercise, our muscles get all stressed. However, in the post-exercise period, they only become stronger as a result of enduring that stress.

In a similar fashion, depriving our bodies of food puts our cells in a stressed state. However, it is only through coping with this stress that these cells become resilient and quickly take up nutrients from the food when we later feed ourselves.

No wonder our adversities make us stronger!

Which takes us to an even more interesting side-effect of IF.

IF triggers a process called 'Cell Autophagy'. To understand this process, let's look at the literal meaning of the word 'Autophagy'. 'Auto' means self and 'phagy' means eat. This translates into self-eating which is essentially what Cell Autophagy is; its when our cells eat themselves up!

Wait, seriously?

Our bodies work in mysterious ways (even though I sound like a broken record saying this again).

However, before you jump the guns and think that there is something wrong with the human species, let me tell you that Cell Autophagy is an evolutionary self-preservation mechanism that is pretty normal and perfectly healthy for our bodies.

If you're still thinking why eating our own body is anything but healthy, you have a very valid point.

And I have a very compelling explanation for you.

When we are eating normally, our cells are preoccupied with dividing and growing without a worry about cleaning any mess that may have built up within themselves. This mess usually comprises any dead or damaged parts of the cell that need to be removed in order to prevent us from some deadly diseases, including cancers.

However, fasting gives a much-needed break to our cells from the normal activities of growth and constant division. These cells, for the lack of a better activity, can now focus on Autophagy which is known to suppress or promote tumors depending on the developmental stage and tumor type.

IF or nutritional restriction is considered one of the most promising techniques to invoke Autophagy, which destroys damaged cells while protecting the normal ones. This can have far reaching implications for chemotherapy as a conventional treatment for cancer, which destroys cancerous cells but is highly toxic to healthy cells at the same time.

Sounds like IF is a rockstar after all!

Ch 3: But That May Not Be All…

While there are some obvious health benefits to IF, are these perks restricted to one's physical health only? As per my knowledge, this isn't the case. I explain precisely why in this chapter.

I know what you must be thinking. There's more?

Yes, my friend. There is!

In the previous sections, we delved into some geeky details of how IF affects a person health-wise. In reality, however, these effects extend far beyond just our physical health.

Come to think of it, some of the benefits of IF we are about to discuss are so unmistakably obvious that you're bound to have an a-ha moment when you read about them.

Sounds too good to be true? Let's see.

Effects for your mental health

A study published in the Neurology International observed the effects of fasting on 29 healthy subjects during Ramadan. These individuals were tested for certain neurotransmitters and neurotrophic factors three times during the research process; 2 days before fasting and on the 14th and 29th day of fasting. The results revealed an increased level of serotonin, brain-derived neurotrophic factor (BDNF), and nerve growth factor (NGF) in the blood of these individuals.

But what does all of this tell us about the impact of fasting on brain health? In simple terms that you and me can understand.

Our neurons, aka brain cells, suffer from a variety of damage and disorders during their lifetime. This can lead to a host of neurological diseases such as Alzheimer's and Parkinson's. Without going much deeper into some incomprehensible details, the neurotransmitters and neurotrophic factors described above play a crucial part in the survival and functioning of these neurons. These neurotrophic factors, also known as neural growth factors (NGF), help repair damaged neurons, thereby preventing neurodegenerative diseases like dementia, Alzheimer's, brain tumors, neuroinfections etc.

Additionally, the Brain-Derived Neurotrophic Factors (BDNF) we talked about earlier not only help our nerve cells survive and thrive but also support the growth of new nerve cells and aid neuronal plasticity; a process through which our brain rewires itself in response to new situations and changes in circumstances it detects.

Studies conducted on rodents show that rats who were fed at certain intervals exhibited better memory and learning than their feasting and partying counterparts. Further research conducted on animals also reveals that IF can help suppress inflammation in the brain, which can otherwise lead to certain neurological conditions and enhance cognitive functions with respect to memory.

However, there is more than one club when it comes to the impact of IF on brain health and wellness. And, to put it simply without stirring too much controversy, it does not support the idea of IF for enhanced mental health.

Those on the other side of the camp contend that IF can lead a person to become hangry (when hunger leads to anger). This is because fasting lowers blood sugar levels and increases cortisol as our cells become stressed due to lack of food. This can lead to mood irritability and may cause people to act more aggressively. Increased cortisol in the system might also make a person more anxious, increase their food cravings and considerably change their food preferences.

Some studies show that fasting can also lower the amount of REM (Rapid Eye Movement aka the deepest and the most restorative phase of one's sleep) due to a decrease in melatonin (a hormone that regulates the sleep-wake cycle). This reduction in melatonin is suspected to be brought about by an increase in cortisol levels which occurs when a person restricts their food intake. The implications are rather self-explanatory; a person who doesn't get a proper night's sleep is bound to feel mentally exhausted during the day and can suffer from an overall degenerative mental health in the long term.

The adversaries of IF also believe that fasting during certain hours of the day may cause a person to skip meals with friends and family which may have a direct impact on their mental health. This is because dining together is considered a strong means of bonding with those that are close to someone, a lack of which is bound to invoke feelings of depression and loneliness.

IF is also believed to facilitate eating disorders in some individuals and change the overall perception of hunger. It is thought to damage our relationship with hunger cues badly, and often permanently, when we ignore them in an attempt to ward off hunger as we fast.

Does this mean that IF does more harm than good when it comes to one's mental health?

While it is a reality that IF may yield some of the negative side effects discussed above, the fact still remains that many of these so-called side effects are actually present when someone just jumps straight into a fast without any prior knowledge or preparation. Cold turkey if you like.

Being hungry and having the hunger pangs keep you up during the night sure doesn't sound that fun, and with the proper preparation, you can honestly reduce the impact of these negative side-effects without too much hassle. Besides, many of these aftereffects of IF subside as a person becomes more accustomed to the practice, and I promise you, the positives definitely outweigh these transient negatives!

Which takes us to the next section.

IF can save you some $$$

IF can be time saving, and time is money, as you might agree.

When you have to worry about only a few meals a day (and not even that sometimes!), then you're bound to save some precious hours on the clock and are free to use this leisure time however you want.

But IF can also save you some actual $$$

Preparing a lesser number of meals implies that you might be able to cut back on your food costs considerably. Although the exact amount of dollar savings you'll get depends on various factors, such as whether you go to an organic store for grocery shopping and how often you enjoy the luxury of dining out, they can be quite sizable when computed on a quarterly or yearly basis.

But since I advocate about healthy eating as much as a sound fasting practice, I'll say that you don't focus too much on how much money you're saving or base your decisions about IF solely on the cost savings involved. As we'll discuss in a later chapter, you might need to make some investments to ensure healthy eating while you're fasting intermittently. And while both of these are two different things, they often complement each other. I'll delve into more detail later, however, at this point I'll only say this.

Whether you save money or spend it on your health, it's a win-win either way!

Effects on circadian rhythm

For those of you thinking that I am throwing fancy terms around yet again, I request to please be patient and bear with me!

A circadian rhythm refers to any physical, mental or behavioral change that follows a pattern. A great example would be feeling sleepy and sluggish during certain hours of the day (think noon and nighttime) while feeling absolutely buzzed and alert at others (say mornings or daytime).

Circadian rhythms are controlled by a part of our brain called the hypothalamus and are affected by external factors such as the amount of daylight in our surroundings. They go beyond just regulating our sleep/wake cycles and effect several other physiological and behavioral changes including metabolism (aka the chemical processes occuring in our bodies to sustain life).

To understand the relationship of fasting with our circadian rhythms and therefore metabolism, let's consider this. According to our evolutionary programming, we are wired to eat during the day and sleep (thereby fast) at night. Our metabolism also performs its best when we let this natural programming guide our routines and don't disrupt it with what plagues the modern society.

However, with trends such as late-night snacking and the hustling culture on the rise, promoting consumption of weird (and often unhealthy) food combinations way past bedtime as well as glorifying working a bizarre number of hours each day, our circadian rhythms are bound to be disrupted taking metabolic efficiency down with them.

Additionally, the effects of these circadian rhythms are less visible when our eating and sleeping patterns are out of whack or when our exposure to daylight is somehow limited or disrupted.

Practicing IF and the time-restricted approach to eating it purports can get our circadian rhythms right back on track. This is because food intake is an effective way to regulate our circadian rhythms, amongst other things. IF allows for an opportunity to align our eating patterns with our biological clock, thereby preserving the precious mechanisms our species has evolved to perfect. When you sleep well, your body's healthy state will naturally follow too.

Hence, not surprisingly, IF is also sometimes called Circadian rhythm fasting.

And rightly so.

Ch 4: Making The Right Choice

What might be best for you

IF can be quite confusing at first with loads of information available on the various approaches one can take to practice it effectively. Which one should you go for? What might best suit you considering your personal state-of-affairs and health conditions? Most importantly, how do you ACTUALLY go about fasting intermittently? Read on to find out!

You might remember that I raved about IF as an immensely flexible practice that can be adapted to suit your particular circumstances and goals.

In other words, no authoritarian diet plans dictating what to eat or not.

This is one of the most compelling aspects of the practice and something that drew me to IF in the first place.

But for someone who has just begun to explore the practice, the various forms of IF they come across can be quite overwhelming which is why this chapter aims to discuss the common methods of fasting intermittently and how they can work for you.

The 16:8 method

This method of practicing IF implies that you fast for 16 hours a day while having an 8-hour window for eating healthy nutritious meals.

If you decide to undertake a 16:8 fast you may, for example, stop eating anything after 7 pm and break your fast at 11 am the next day. One can, however, consume water and other calorie-free drinks such as black tea and coffee during the fasting period.

The 16:8 method of IF is ideal for individuals who want to lose weight and aim to incorporate IF in their daily routines without any major disruptions. This is because all you have to do is plan an early dinner, which is something that a lot of folks with families and young kids already prefer, and then delay breakfast a little to practice a 16:8 fast.

Additionally, this method does not demand an immense amount of self-control since much of the fasting period would be spent sleeping. With time, a 16:8 fast can curb your desire to eat late into the evenings or snack as long as you're awake at night, making it even more convenient to practice IF this way.

The 16:8 fast is considered one of the most sustainable forms of IF which is why you mustn't worry about being unable to continue it in the long term. Studies suggest that it not only helps people lose weight but also reduces the systolic blood pressure and improves the overall health of an individual.

Nonetheless, some dieticians recommend that people who are on a high-carb diet should be wary of the 16:8 method. This is because a diet high in carbs induces increased insulin levels. When a person fasts, these high insulin levels can cause hypoglycemia (low blood sugar levels). The same goes for people on medication for diabetes and diuretic drugs.

In short, while it is an ideal start for people dipping their toes into IF, those individuals with any complex health conditions must consult their physicians before embarking on the 16:8 bandwagon.

The 5:2 method

Being yet another relatively flexible form of IF, the 5:2 method advocates that you eat normally 5 days a week and consume no more than 500-600 calories on your fasting days. You can feast or fast on any day of your preference so long as you keep the 5:2 schedule in mind and sandwich at least one non-fasting day in between your fasts.

The 5:2 method is particularly beneficial for individuals who find it hard to practice a certain IF regimen throughout the week and speculate that two days of calorie-managed eating could work equally well for them.

With the 5:2 method, there are no strict rules when it comes to consuming food during fasting days except minding the calorie restriction. However, it is critical that you not only be mindful of the amount of calories consumed while fasting but also the type of calories you are consuming on your restricted days in order to make the most of your calorie-budget.

It is recommended, therefore, that you eat food that is highly nutritious and high in fiber as well as protein. This will ensure that you feel full early without having to eat much.

The 5:2 method of IF has shown to have some impressive health benefits, including but not limited to weight loss, lower insulin resistance and a decrease in inflammation.

Nonetheless, it is not suitable for individuals with a history of eating disorders or for those who are prone to hypoglycemia. Additionally, pregnant or nursing mothers, type-1 diabetics, malnourished or underweight individuals and children as well as women struggling with fertility issues should avoid it or consult with their physician before having a go at it.

The time-restricted method

Since we are all about flexibility and convenience here, let's talk about another method of practicing IF that allows for even more leeway!

The time-restricted method.

As the name implies, this method of IF gives you the freedom to choose your eating window every.single.day. (with ideally a 14-16 hour fasting period)

To make it even easier, you can adjust your eating window such that most of the fasting time is spent sleeping and will therefore fly by you without you even realizing it.

Beware, nonetheless, that the timing of the fasting window has to be set so as to trigger ketosis (we covered ketosis in detail in one of the previous chapters) which normally kicks in after 12 hours and is full-blown effective after 14-16 hours of eating nothing.

In addition to initializing ketosis, the time-restricted method flaunts all the usual benefits associated with IF in general; weight loss as well as a lower insulin resistance and inflammation in the body.

This method of practicing IF is particularly suitable for individuals with constantly varying schedules or for those that have to travel frequently since it will allow these folks to adjust their eating and fasting windows as and when needed. Besides, this form of IF can also work well for newbies who are still experimenting with IF and are still on the lookout for an ideal time to fast.

The whole-day fasting method

The whole-day fasting method is exactly what it seems. It involves fasting for a full 24 hours, usually once or twice a week, while eating normally for the rest of the week. During the fasting period, one can have water, tea and other calorie-free drinks but no food.

Depending on your preference, you can fast from one meal to the other; be that breakfast, lunch or dinner.

Whatever fancies you.

This regimen is considered quite impactful for weight loss but can cause headaches, fatigue or irritability in individuals who aren't accustomed to IF or fasting for extended periods of time in general. It is, therefore, recommended that you first try a lighter version of IF such as the 16:8 method to let your body acclimatize to abstinence before working your way up to full day fasts.

The whole-day fasting regimen is not suitable for someone who suffers from a complicated health condition such as hypoglycemia, which is why such people must consult their physician before attempting to fast for 24 hours straight.

The alternate-day fasting method

As the name suggests, alternate-day fasting involves fasting every other day. This type of fasting can take one of the two forms; you can either fast completely and consume no calories whatsoever on the fasting day or restrict yourself to one meal consisting of about 500 calories while fasting.

Quite a famous regimen for weight loss, alternate-day fasting can be really challenging to sustain in the long term. The reason is simple; it is difficult to fast every other day for the majority of people. Additionally, while this form of IF is proven by research to create noticeable weight loss in the first 8-12 weeks, its efficacy wanes as more time passes. This is because consistent alternate-day fasting can lead to increased calorie intake during the non-fasting days, ultimately setting off any weight loss that might have been achieved while fasting.

Alternate-day fasting is not endorsed for individuals with any serious and complicated health condition and for those who are just beginning to explore IF since it can easily scare newbies away.

OMAD

Otherwise known as One meal a day.

Yep, you heard me. Practitioners of this method actually just consume a meal on a daily basis. Now, before you jump to conclusions about not having sufficient nutritional intake and all those perfectly legitimate concerns, let me just say that folks who do OMAD are usually seasoned practitioners of intermittent fasting.

What that means is that their bodies are already tuned to the fasting hours and they are perfectly enjoying perks that IF brings to them. That is also part of the reason why they can take the step up to do OMAD.

As scary as it sounds having just one meal a day, the actual caloric intake may not differ that much from someone who is practicing the 16:8 method in actuality. OMAD in its essential form is just a lengthening of the fasting window, and consequently a shortening of the feasting timeframe.

This gives the body more time without food, as well as the impact of food, so that it can perform all those wonderful stuff like ketosis and autophagy without interruption.

OMAD will take some getting used to, and not everyone will be able to conscientiously practice it, but for those who manage to do it, the benefits are definitely more than just reducing the time you need to eat and cook!

Fasting as you will!

Let's admit it: after going through all the various forms of IF above, this much can be said in confidence;

This s*** is flexible as hell!

But did you know that you'd still be practicing a particular form of IF if you just paid close attention to your hunger cues and ate only when your body desired?

Yeah. I wasn't fooling around with you!

The fasting as you will method of IF can be interpreted however you like, so long as you can be sensitive to the hunger cues your body sends you. While the exact regimen you build out of this depends on your own particular needs, it broadly encompasses eating mindfully almost all the time, allowing for fasting for extended periods of time and treating yourself occasionally for your good behavior.

It is usually a smart approach to involve your physician while doing this in order to ensure that you're not overplaying it and to prevent yourself from damaging your health or aggravating an already existing health condition.

This form of IF is particularly beneficial for individuals who have a hard time following a fixed schedule or for those who would like to take a short break from any of the IF methods described above. After all, it's a reality of life; things don't always go like you would want them to. Which is why the fasting as you will approach can come in handy when you find yourself basking in the sun in the Bahamas or when a close family member is getting married and you can't be less bothered about a fasting regimen.

The key thing about fasting as you will is the noticing of your hunger cues. The trick here is to focus on real hunger and not perceived hunger. We know by now that our modern age has created a sugar glut and consequently shifted our body's response to food. We are craving more food even as we tuck in to the empty calories of sugar laden processed grub. In that kind of situation, wanting to do fasting as you will definitely will not work. What should be done would be to acclimatize the body with the easier 16:8 so as to restore the body's natural hunger cues, and then this method of IF would be more feasible in practice.

Now that we are familiar with almost all of the major methods of practicing IF, let's examine exactly how one is supposed to embark on an IF journey, regardless of the approach they take.

Ch 5: Step By Step

How to get started?

"Beginnings are the hardest but worth it in the end"

-Unknown

With the spirit of the above quote in mind, let's begin a step-by-step guide for exactly how to fast intermittently.

Step 1: Get clear on your goals

Having clear goals can take you far in life generally, but don't underestimate the importance of defining your objectives before you begin an IF regimen.

For me, it was losing the excess weight I had put on during and after pregnancy (this consequently solved a bunch of other health issues for me), improving metabolic health as well as achieving mental sharpness and focus. Broadly speaking, I wanted to experience an overall better health for my own sake, and most importantly, my baby's. However, my research indicated that I needed to define exactly what I wanted out of IF in order to reap its full benefits.

And let me explain why this is the case.

Defining your goals when it comes to IF is critical for a number of reasons. First and foremost, it allows you to pick the most suitable IF method that will effectively take you closer to what you want. For instance, the Alternate-Day IF method is more fitting for those aiming to lose weight while the 16:8 method is more of a healthy lifestyle change.

While weight loss is one of the most popular reasons people embark on an IF journey, you might have your own reasons for giving IF a chance. Find out what you want out of the practice and then move to step 2 below.

Step 2: Choose your method

Now that you know exactly what you're seeking from IF, the next step involves picking a suitable IF method that will help you achieve your goals.

You can choose from any of the methods of IF described at the beginning of this chapter depending on your goals, personal preferences and health conditions.

In addition to your specific goals regarding IF, there are other factors that also go into choosing an IF method that would yield the most benefits for you. These include the length of time you want to fast for, your daily routine, what field of work you're employed in and what a typical workday looks like for you, the specific climatic conditions prevailing in your part of the world and how often you dine out with friends and family, to name a few.

Once you have chosen an IF method, though, remember that you're not stuck with it forever. It is completely possible to transition from one type of IF to another if you find that your current regimen isn't working for you or if you think you've mastered the moderate forms of IF (think 16:8 method) and want to go pro and explore some relatively challenging routes such as the Alternate-Day fasting.

Besides, it is advisable for a person to give at least one month's serious go to any particular IF method before quitting or switching it up for good.

Step 3: identify your calorie needs

Now that you know what you want from IF and how you're going to approach it, the next step involves finding a way to figure out and manage your calories. This is important because if your top goal for IF is weight loss, then you need to consume less calories than you burn for energy i.e. build a calorie-deficit. While IF is naturally designed to create a calorie deficit when you're fasting, this can be quickly turned into a surplus if you're not mindful of the calories you consume during your eating windows.

Some people practicing IF are usually the least concerned about counting and measuring the calories they consume. Although keeping track of one's calorie consumption is important to a certain extent (even while fasting intermittently), these folks are of the opinion that their calorie consumption is automatically taken care of as a direct result of fasting intermittently. While this may work out well for someone who doesn't suffer from (or is prone to) an eating disorder such as Anorexia, Orthorexia and Binge eating, it can be detrimental for individuals whose eating disorders may be triggered by IF.

Keeping a track of the amount of calories you consume during IF is also important because even if certain methods of IF such as the Alternate-Day fasting do allow for calorie consumption during fasting days, there is a limit to how much of these calories one can consume. Again, this restriction is meant to facilitate the benefits of IF such as weight loss.

Besides, there is a popular opinion that as long as you consume just under 50 calories in the morning, you will be considered to be in the fasted state. This can be critical for those practicing the 16:8 method by having an early dinner and delayed breakfast in an attempt to reach a 16-hour milestone with their fasting. Such people can drink plain water or have a cup of black coffee (no added sugar!) without the risk of breaking their fast in the mornings.

But, guess what, this also implies that you have to be mindful of the calories you consume in order to make sure that your IF regimen is not put to waste.

All of this leads to one conclusion only: whether you're fasting or feasting, you must keep an eye on your calorie consumption in order to achieve your goals with IF. At least in the beginning.

Nowadays, there are a variety of apps that can be used to track calorie intake. Some of the best ones include MyFitnessPal and Lose It! which not only include a calorie counter but also boasts a food diary and an exercise log.

As you get the hang of doing IF in any shape or form that you think best suits you and your situation, the focus on calorie intake will usually wind up fading into the background as IF and your new eating habits get ingrained into your schedule. You will find that you do not need to track the calories as much because you know the approximate amounts which you consume on a daily basis. This is when the much vaunted benefit of not needing to calorie count comes back straight into play, with a vengeance! Because you have more practice and have already established a fair routine and habit doing your IF lifestyle, your daily caloric intake is more or less at your fingertips. Consequently, you end up not having to pay too much attention to that, and can carry on with your daily stuff without having to worry about the calorie count.

Step 4: Conduct meal planning (without overdoing it!)

And no. I'm not about to contradict myself here.

We discussed earlier that IF is quite liberating in the sense that it allows one to let go of the tedious job of meal planning all the time.

And I'm not going back on my words here.

This step is, in fact, pretty optional. You can choose to do it, or not.

IF is not a practice meant to put restrictions on someone when it comes to what they eat.

Nonetheless, we all know that a balanced and nutritious diet is critical for maintaining good health, regardless of whether or not you practice IF.

One thing that must be understood is that restricting food for a certain number of hours does not justify consuming junk food when the eating window finally opens. Making unhealthy food choices when you finally sit down to eat in an IF regimen is not only detrimental for your overall health but will also put any and all of your efforts with regards to IF go to waste.

And you don't want that.

Therefore, it is recommended that you take some time out to (informally) plan what you will eat during say, the week ahead. This will not help you keep track of your calorie intake (and thereby lose and maintain weight consistently) but also ensure that you have everything you need to cook a healthy, nutritious and delicious meal on hand (we will discuss an effective and easy way of meal-prepping later in the book).

Because, let's be honest, we are more susceptible to ordering takeaway food and eating unhealthy snacks when prepping a healthy meal at home becomes difficult due to any reason.

And frankly, if you find yourself eating loads of unhealthy food when you aren't fasting, you might as well not fast at all!

Step 5: Begin your IF journey with the pedal to the metal!

Once you have completed all of the steps above, you are now ready to begin your IF journey and see where it takes you.

Along with all of my very best wishes, here are a few things that I would like you to keep in mind while you're at it:

- Make the calories count in the beginning by keeping the nutritional value of any food you consume in sight
- Practice moderation, both while fasting and feasting
- Take IF as an opportunity to improve your eating habits and food choices. Less meals mean more time for preparing healthy food to dine on!
- IF isn't a one-size-fits-all approach so keep experimenting to figure out what works best for you!

Ch 6: Eating And Fasting

Re-learning eating

IF is a lifestyle change and to ensure your success with the practice, you might have to re-learn some of your eating habits. This chapter walks you through how to do this important task while fasting intermittently. All the best!

Although IF does not explicitly put any restrictions on what you should eat or avoid consuming altogether, it won't do harm to follow some general guidelines for eating nonetheless.

In fact, these recommendations are only meant to enhance the health benefits you might expect from following an IF regimen.

This is, in part, loosely related to identifying your calorie needs as covered in the previous chapter. However, this chapter focuses more on the types of food you should prefer consuming while fasting intermittently instead of counting the calories you're putting in your body.

Don't get confused. Both of these things are important in their own right.

It's just that our focus here is a little different, that's all.

As we discussed previously as well, making unhealthy food choices during one's eating windows may offset any health benefits they were bound to receive during fasting, such as weight loss. This emphasizes the fact that while eating healthy is always important, it is critical to garner the most out of an IF regimen, unless you want to treat yourself occasionally.

Besides, IF does allow you to consume certain foods during fasting, without facing the risk of breaking your fast.

So, what exactly is recommended? Nothing fancy, if you ask me.

Just a typical rundown of what healthy eating normally constitutes with a focus on IF.

It is common knowledge that not all foods are created equal when it comes to their nutritious value. This brings us to the following list of edibles you can safely consume, both during and after the fasting periods, in order to ensure that you're getting the maximum out of your IF regimen.

Foods to eat while fasting

While fasting implies an abstinence from food, there are certain things that you can still devour without putting a dent in your regimen.

Here are some of those more forgiving foods:

- Plain old water: Thankfully, your good ol' friend water steers clear of the no-go area. You can consume plain water or diet versions of the tonic water to keep yourself hydrated during a fast without adding to the calorie count.

- Tea and coffee: both tea and coffee (without added sugar, milk or cream) can be consumed during a fast. Black coffee might actually enhance the benefits of IF since it is demonstrated to support healthy blood sugar levels over the long term.

- Apple cider vinegar (diluted): apple cider vinegar can be consumed during fasting as well as eating windows. Along with its antimicrobial and antioxidant properties, ACV can enhance the benefits of IF by supporting healthy blood sugar and digestion as well as keeping a person hydrated during a fast.

- Bone broth: A bone (or veggie) broth is highly recommended during IF as it supplies the body with essential amino acids as well as other minerals and vitamins while instilling a feeling of being full. However, be highly aware of canned or store-bought varieties of broth that contain a shitload of artificial flavors and preservatives. Instead, stir up a nice homemade broth with a little bit of seasalt to promote water retention during fasting.

- Healthy fats: while this one may seem obviously controversial, consuming healthy fats such as MCT oil, ghee, butter and coconut oil can support ketosis. Granted, these will technically break your fast. However, they can also help you survive the rest of the fasting period without relying on some unhealthy carbs that will put the precious ketosis to an end.

Foods to eat when you're not fasting

While you may think that the world is yours once your fasting period ends, remember that it is always a good practice to be mindful of what you are putting in your body in order to build on the benefits of fasting you just banked on.

I may sound like a broken record saying this repeatedly...

But ya' friend can't emphasize this point enough.

The last thing you want to do is spoil everything you've just earned through fasting by gobbling a huge slice(s) of pizza or feeding on an extra-large burger with fries.

Sounds tempting...

Ain't recommended though.

What's more, fasting intermittently means that you have a relatively narrower eating window than normal. If you don't eat well during these windows of opportunity, you might put yourself at the risk of facing malnutrition that can lead to a host of undesirable health conditions.

Eating after you've fasted for a considerable amount of time can be challenging in a few ways. Not only do you have to ensure that you're eating nutrient-dense food but you must also be cautious of putting too much too soon on your digestive system.

Which is why I'm including a list of foods that you can refer to when the time comes to finally eat something:

- Healthy fats: breaking your fast with healthy fats such as coconut and olive oil, avocados, eggs, ghee and grass-fed butter will ensure that your digestive system is not overwhelmed and that you get the right nutrients that your body craves for after a fast.

- Soups: soups and broths aren't only good when you're fasting but can also be a great source of nutrients and vitamins when you're finally ready to eat again. While a simple veggie or bone broth can be your best friend during fasting, you can add a bunch of stuff like lentils, tofu or pasta to spice it up for the post-fasting period.

- Veggies: most of us don't need another long and boring lesson on the importance of consuming vegetables, but here it is again (I promise to keep it short though!). While all veggies are good for health, some starchy ones such as sweet potatoes can be a great source of resistant starches when breaking a fast. Just make sure that you cook them up thoroughly.

- Smoothies: these are a great way to give your body the nutrient-punch it needs after fasting for several hours. What's more, smoothies are always fun to make since you can throw together almost anything and stir up a nutritious yet delicious drink within minutes. Not a vegetable person? Add in some romaine lettuce or spinach in your blend in order to prevent missing out on the benefits of these leafy greens without having to consume a bowl full of baked veggies instead.

- Fermented foods: foods such as unsweetened yogurt and kefir are a great source of probiotics that your gut is going to thank you over a million times for. Yogurt also contains almost all the nutrients that our bodies need, including but not limited to, calcium, B vitamins, proteins, phosphorus and vitamin D. It is a precious source of trace minerals and is found to be particularly beneficial for osteoporosis and digestive health.

- Fruits (fresh & dried): to keep it light on your gut, you can also break your fast with fruits such as watermelon, grapes and honeydew. These are ideal because they contain a high water-content to combat dehydration and are easily digestible. If you want some inspiration from folks in other parts of the world then don't look beyond the Middle-East and Arabia. People inhabiting these regions prefer to break their fasts with dates which are a dense source of nutrients and restore energy levels after a long fast. If dates are not your thing, try dried apricots or raisins for similar effects.

The above guide can be extremely helpful when one finally finds themselves in the eating window because it is pretty easy to get carried away by all those hunger pangs and eat whatever comes your way. However, I can guarantee from personal experience that if you let yourself indulge at that point, then you're going to regret it later.

It only takes a few minutes of mindless eating to come back to your senses and realize that you've just spoiled everything you worked for till that point.

The meal planning thing we discussed earlier is all the more important for this reason; when you don't know what kind of healthy meal awaits you at the end of your fast, you're more prone to eating whatever comes your way regardless of the consequences.

The end result may look something like this:

Snacking ---→ Guilt ---→ Binge-Eating ---→ More Guilt (and the cycle continues on to more snacking)

You definitely do not want that.

Supplements and IF

If you're somehow against supplements or haven't considered taking them before, you are missing out on something extremely important for maintaining good health.

In his book 'The Plant Paradox', Dr. Steven R. Gundry explains that he is a convert when it comes to supplements. There was a time that Dr. Gundry used to perceive supplements as useless pills that did nothing but produce colorful urine. However, what dramatically altered the perceptions of this highly successful physician and heart surgeon was a study of the effects of vitamins, minerals and nutrients on the biomarkers of inflammation in his patients.

In his book, Dr. Gundry cites the actual wording in the U.S Senate Document to emphasize the importance of supplements. The said document explicitly states that the produce we currently consume lacks in important nutrients because the land used to cultivate it is no longer rich with these nutrients in the first place.

While this piece of information is a revelation in itself, what is even more surprising is the origin of this document, which dates as far back as 1936!

These scientists knew that we couldn't meet all of our nutritional needs by relying on the consumption of food alone, no matter how healthy it might be, AND they knew it way earlier than one could imagine.

While supplements are necessary for everyone, they can be extremely beneficial for those fasting intermittently since they are at a higher risk for failing to meet their body's nutritional needs. This is particularly true when undergoing prolonged periods of fasting and consuming a relatively unhealthy and non-nutritious diet when not.

However, should you decide to include dietary supplements in your daily routine or are already taking them, there are certain things to keep in mind when it comes to IF.

Certain supplements are more likely to break a fast than others. Care to know what these are?

Supplements to AVOID while fasting

- Gummy vitamins-contain sugar, protein and fat
- Protein powders-contain calories
- BCAAs (Branch Chain Amino Acids)-can raise insulin levels thereby putting a stop to ketosis and oppose autophagy
- Any fat soluble vitamins that are best taken with meals

Supplements you CAN take while fasting

- Multivitamins- those without added sugars and fillers
- Creatine
- Collagen- may slightly impact autophagy
- Probiotics and prebiotics

- Individual supplements for certain nutrients such as Vitamin A & D, zinc and copper- some of these are best taken with a meal though!
- Fish (or algae) oil- contains few calories

So far, the above discussion establishes this much; what you eat matters, whether you're fasting or not and that it is all the more important to be mindful of your diet while fasting intermittently.

Also, let's not forget that supplementation is important for our health.

However, our health is not entirely dependent on diet and supplements, it also requires that we maintain a certain lifestyle that will ensure our well being in the long term. This lifestyle encompasses physical activity, weight and stress management as well as healthy eating.

In other words, being physically and mentally healthy for the long haul not only demands that we eat healthy but also requires that we remain physically active and manage our stress levels.

And exercise is a critical part of the physical activity and stress management equation.

But how does one go about following their workout routine with considerably long periods of fasting throughout a day?

Take it from me, the upcoming section adequately covers the above question.

Exercising and fasting intermittently

Come to think of it, IF is more of a lifestyle change. For instance, when you expect to wake up and skip breakfast on purpose, this could mean a lot for how you spend the rest of the day (eating and otherwise).

Continuing with the same train of thought, it is only natural that IF will impact the activities you conduct in a typical day, including exercise. And for those of you who hold their workout routines near and dear to their hearts, this could mean a lot.

While exercising during IF is not entirely beyond the bounds of possibility, it depends on a number of factors such as what time of the day you normally do your workouts and how your body feels at the time. The most important thing to understand is that you might need to adjust your workout routine with your IF regimen (or vice versa) in order to come up with a plan that works best for you.

Don't forget that IF is quite a forgiving regimen and that you can use this flexibility to your advantage. I'll go into more details of how to do so in a minute but before that let's examine if there are any benefits to working out on an empty stomach.

One of the most bragged about advantages of exercising in a fasted state is that it promotes fat burning. As we discussed earlier as well, glycogen (aka glucose) from carbs is the primary source of fuel that our body utilizes for energy production. When fasting intermittently, this much-loved source of fuel is already on the lower side, allowing our body to burn fat for energy (Remember ketosis?). Therefore, when working out on an empty stomach, there is a higher chance that you will burn fat in the absence of glucose.

And who doesn't want that?

Not quite surprisingly, there is a flip side to this situation as well.

When our body finds out that glycogen isn't available, it might also turn towards breaking down protein (muscle) for fueling itself during an intense workout. Now this is a matter of concern because you want to lose fat not muscle. And while you're obviously losing some fat while working out in the absence of glycogen, your muscle mass is on the line as well.

Besides, intensive workouts in the absence of carbs (or other sources of calories) to burn as fuel may also lead to slower metabolism in the long run. When the body discovers that there aren't any calories accessible to consume for energy, it slows the metabolism in an attempt to manage calorie consumption in anticipation of a potential fuel crisis. A slower metabolism isn't good. It can cause all sorts of health issues such as unexplained weight gain or difficulty losing weight, chronic fatigue, skin, hair & nail issues as well as depression and constipation.

Now that that's out of the way, let's discuss how you can adapt your workout routine in accordance with the IF regimen you're following (or vice versa) in order to gain the maximum benefit for your health and to keep any potential harm at bay. It is also recommended that you prefer modifying your IF regimen in the light of your workout routine (instead of the other way around) in order to avoid disrupting a habit that's already established. This is because not only is it hard to build a habit in the first place, it can be a real challenge to work on founding two of them at a time.

The most sought after question in this regard remains this:

Should I workout during the fasting or eating window?

The answer to this question isn't quite straightforward. It all depends on what method of IF you're currently following and what goals you want to achieve with your workout routine.

With that being said, the above discussion on the pros and cons of exercising while fasting intermittently should give you some perspective on how to approach this matter.

According to experts, your take on the above question will vary significantly depending on why you're working out in the first place. If you're someone whose sole purpose of training is to reap some general health benefits without much focus on athletic performance, then you can exercise during the eating or fasting window, whichever suits you and aligns with how you feel at that particular time.

On the contrary, if you're someone who has an intensive workout routine that aims to enhance competitive performance, the timing of your exercise and eating becomes much more relevant.

For instance, those following the 16:8 method of IF and working out for weight loss and general fitness can continue their morning workouts in a fasted state and wait for the lunchtime to get themselves fed. On the other hand, folks that are strength training for the purpose of enhancing athletic performance can consider modifying their IF hours to allow for an early lunch. This could mean, for example, having dinner a bit earlier than scheduled (7pm instead of 8pm) so they can break their fast early (11 am the next day).

This must be considered in conjunction with the discussion we had in the beginning of this section. A more intense workout implies that you need more energy. If you haven't fueled yourself up right before, say an intensive cardio lineup, you are more prone to breaking down muscle mass along with fat.

It also brings us to another popular concern when it comes to exercising while fasting intermittently; whether one should eat before exercise or schedule grub right after working out. Again, this depends on your goals for the workout routine you're following as well as how your body feels about exercising in a fasted state.

But before I present any more guidance on this subject, I would like you to consider the concept of an 'Anabolic Window'. An anabolic window refers to a post-exercise period of about 30 minutes during which any consumption of proteins and carbs can aid the growth of muscle mass. This can be particularly crucial for people who are strength training since they can support muscle growth by timing the consumption of carbs and proteins right after an intensive workout session.

Not so much for the other folks though.

People who exercise for general health and fitness need not worry much about the anabolic window. Such individuals can eat before or after a workout depending on how they feel. This implies that each one of us has to experiment in order to figure out what'll work for us realistically.

Have you noticed how calorie consumption while working out during IF is completely contextual?

You can approach it in a number of ways.

And while we're still talking about ways, let's discuss another method to manage eating before (or after) exercise.

This approach involves consuming more calories on days when you're having a rather intensive training schedule than others. It is known as 'carb cycling' and implies that you eat plenty of carbs on days when you're supposed to do an intensive workout and go easy on the ones when you're resting or doing light exercises. This will not only allow you to build muscle on days when you're going all-out but will also help promote fat loss when you're consuming lesser carbs on other casual days.

Think all of this information is a little mind-boggling? If you could take just one thing away from the above discussion, it could be this:

The relation between your IF regimen and workout routine is highly dependent on your training goals and personal experiences. These can be adjusted to garner the maximum benefit from both your IF regimen and workout routine with a little thought and experimentation.

Before we move on to the next chapter and wind this one up for good, let me share with you a few things to keep in mind with regard to your workout routine while fasting intermittently. Consider it a sort of rundown for whatever we've discussed above as well as a few bonus tips to keep in mind when you're heading for the gym.

- The type of IF regimen you're following will have a direct impact on your workout routine. Don't expect to ace your high-intensity interval training when fasting for a full day

- Try to stay in the 'safe' zone. Don't push yourself too hard and listen closely to what your body has to tell you. For instance, when feeling weak or dizzy during those lunges, skip 'em and go for something lighter like a walk

- Match your nutrient intake with your workout. Both the timing and nutritional value is of importance here

- High-intensity strength training requires more carbs to be consumed within the same day (reminder: consider 'carb recycling' discussed above). It is recommended that you schedule your more intensive training sessions as close to your last meal as possible

- If you're aiming to build muscle mass, you should schedule your IF routine such that there is a pre-workout snack planned as well as a meal rich in proteins for right after. While the pre-workout snack will provide the fuel for training, the post-workout proteins are meant to help your muscles repair and grow after an intensive drill

- At the end of the day, if you're eating enough nutritious food during the eating windows, there isn't much to worry about (strength training is a different story though!)

- Try to keep yourself hydrated in the fasting window with plain water (or coconut water for a boost of electrolytes)

- There is no one-size-fits-all approach. The fasting and exercising regimen will differ for everyone out there. Keep experimenting and find out what works best for you

Ch 7: The How-To & Not-To

Everybody makes mistakes

We as humans are bound to make mistakes. The same goes for an IF regimen whose flexibility makes it more prone to people making some serious blunders all the time. What are these and how to avoid them? Let's find out!

As I am writing these words, the people in my country and everyone else on the globe are fighting the Coronavirus disease aka the infamous Covid-19. Many countries have been forced to significantly reduce their activities with regard to work, education and leisure while some nations such as Italy are facing lockdown. As research on this novel coronavirus carries on and new information unfolds every hour, this is something that undoubtedly has everybody scared witless.

And yes, it is Covid-19, the virus itself that has become a nightmare for all of us.

But what is even more alarming is the uncertainty surrounding this new disease which is now declared a pandemic.

And in the wake of these confusing (and extremely dangerous) times, everybody is making their own mistakes and learning from them.

And while talking about Covid-19 and how it is spreading all over the world around us calls for another book solely dedicated to the topic, my point is that it is natural for us to make mistakes and learn from them as we go, particularly when we aren't certain about the best course of action.

The same applies to IF.

While there is extensive guidance available on how to approach IF, we can all make mistakes sometimes. This is especially relevant since IF allows a significant amount of wiggle room for experimentation, implying that people may be making some mistakes with regard to the practice, although unintentionally.

Now, I understand that those just embarking on their IF journey are bound to make some slips. However, these common blunders can sometimes be made by experts as well.

What are these? Let's find out together.

Doing too much too soon

This one, in particular, applies to both beginners and pros. Let me explain how.

When I began intermittent fasting for the first time, I was excited, to say the least. In fact, ya' girl was so pumped by all the information her research had yielded that she wanted to fast for 24 hours straight (with only water and black tea allowed in between).

The result?

If you haven't guessed it already, I gave up after the first day!

The biggest mistake I made as a naive IF beginner was thinking I could go all in without letting my body become accustomed to fasting for shorter periods of time first.

Unfortunately, I was gravely mistaken. But fortunately, I was determined to make it work. Therefore I figured that something needed to be changed if I was to continue fasting intermittently.

And that is exactly what I'll recommend to you.

Our bodies are used to the normal eating patterns we have established over the years. This involves eating three meals a day and grabbing on a snack whenever the craving for one arises. So when you suddenly skip on breakfast and plan a 16-hour fast, your body is bound to retaliate.

And this retaliation can express itself in the form of low blood-glucose levels, lethargy, some seriously painful hunger pangs and mood irritability, to name a few.

Honestly, were you expecting something else?

But there is a solution.

Physicians recommend giving your body the time it needs to get used to this new eating routine. This can be done by, for example, aiming to achieve a 12-hour gap between breakfast and dinner in the beginning and then gradually stretching this gap. Besides, you can always start with the 16:8 method of IF which is considered the most beginner-friendly. Plan an early dinner (say 7 pm) and try not to have breakfast until 11 am the next day. This way, most of your fasting time will be spent sleeping and you won't have to face the unpleasant side effects of IF.

What we've discussed so far was mostly relevant to beginners. However, the pros also make the same mistake, albeit in a slightly different manner. For instance, a person who has been practicing the 16:8 method for a few weeks might think that they can transition to a full 24-hour fast twice a week. If this individual is not careful about ensuring that this transition is made gradually (say, extending the 16-hour fast by 2 hours every week), they are putting themselves at a serious risk of facing all the negative side effects we talked about earlier.

Your body needs time to adjust to fasting intermittently, don't push it too hard or you'll cause it to work for the side of giving up! We know we can use all the help we can get while fasting intermittently, do it gradually and let our bodies be in on our side as well.

Sucking the joy out of it!

IF is meant to be a flexible regimen that can be adapted to your particular needs and circumstances. If you try to make it work like it's something set in stone then it might not be sustainable for long term.

I was just two months into IF when some of my friends planned a weekend-long getaway. Work had us all chained up really bad at that time and a few of us weren't even in the same state anymore. As you could imagine, we were genuinely looking forward to this weekend retreat in order to break free from our daily routines and had done everything in our power to clear our schedules.

Amidst all this excitement, I completely forgot that I was following an IF regimen that I needed to stick to and that won't allow me to enjoy the elaborate breakfasts, assorted lunches and amazing martinis we had planned for our trip. Long story short, while others in the group were partying hard and having the time of their lives, I found myself avoiding the fun with a sullen mood that lasted almost the entire trip.

Lesson of the day: make room for when you're having fun with your friends and (for a short while) forget that you have a regimen to follow!

If you are constantly turning down dinner invites and avoiding family get-togethers in order to keep up with your IF regimen then you'll soon be frustrated and might abandon IF completely. A better solution is to use the flexibility IF offers to create some form of leeway for yourself so that you can enjoy social minglings while continuing with IF at the same time.

The next time someone invites you to a dinner party, why not move your lunch time further along in the upcoming day to compensate for that late-night baked chicken and beef stew?

Shouldn't be that much of a problem, right?

Choosing the method that doesn't go with your lifestyle

Some people go into IF without realizing that it is a lifestyle change that will have considerable impact on other areas of their life. Besides eating.

To give you some perspective, if someone does high-intensity training first thing in the morning, then it is a bad idea for them to skip breakfast or a pre-workout snack. Or if one has a night job that keeps them up until dawn it would be impractical for them to have an early dinner and hope to break their fast with lunch the next day. That is simply not viable!

My advice is not to put yourself into unnecessary trouble by choosing an IF regimen that contradicts with how you normally go about your day. Because if you do so, you're setting yourself up for some real headache.

Exploiting the eating window

This one is true for so many people practicing IF (including the beginner-me!). Yes, I was guilty of making all sorts of bad food choices when the eating window finally opened its dear arms to me.

The end result was nothing but sheer disappointment in myself and the self-control I possessed.

This is probably the biggest paradox of an IF regimen; it puts a limit to when you can eat but not on what you should eat. This otherwise valuable facet of IF is often interpreted as we just have to wait for the fasting period to end in order to eat whatever we're craving.

But this attitude is risky for a few important reasons. First and foremost (and as we discussed earlier as well), eating non-nutritious food when you aren't fasting puts everything you've worked for so far to waste. Secondly, this mindset of exploiting the eating window can lead to overeating or binge-eating, both of which can tip the scales against the weight loss benefits of IF. And last but not the least, how you tend to utilize your eating windows can have a direct impact on your fasting experience.

Confused about this final one? Let me explain.

Whatever we provide our bodies as fuel in the form of food, they use it for energy production. Similar to cars, this can be either premium-grade gasoline or diesel (the latter doesn't burn as clean as the former). We discussed earlier that our main source of energy is glucose from carbs. However, an increased carb reliance can make fasting a bit of a challenge because glucose is readily burned by the body for fuel, spikes our blood sugar levels and makes our appetite fluctuate constantly. On the contrary, a low-carb diet with an emphasis on fats and proteins can keep one full for longer and thereby make fasting easier.

And once your body is in a position to fast for longer periods of time, you can expect it to switch successfully to alternative sources of fuel such as fat. The ketones that are obtained as a result of burning fat aren't only cleaner but a more efficient source of energy. And being in ketosis mode implies that your IF regimen is already working out.

Isn't that killing two birds with one stone?

Therefore, you must be mindful of what you put in your body when you aren't fasting. A good way to do that is to plan ahead for the week and have a healthy and nutritious meal scheduled for every day. This might sound a bit tedious at first but will ensure that you eat healthy all-week-long and are set free from the trouble of meal planning for an entire week at the same time.

Not so bad if you factor in the benefits, right?

Starving yourself, even after fasting

Interestingly, while it is completely possible to exploit your eating window by consuming more than you're supposed to, it is also highly likely that you may be starving yourself even when you're finally allowed to eat.

I interpret this in two ways since there is more than one unique approach to starving yourself. The first one is apparent; you aren't eating enough to meet your body's nutritional needs. I'm referring to the quantity of your food servings here. The other one points towards starving yourself when you aren't consuming enough nutrient-dense food during the eating window and are consuming a lot of empty calories that are simply filling the stomach.

Which is, quite frankly, equivalent to starving yourself.

This is bad for obvious reasons; your body's nutritional needs remain unmet, your muscle mass is put at risk and your metabolic rate may slow down over the long term.

However, another major danger associated with starvation is that you're ultimately putting yourself at a higher risk of what I call an eating-ricochet. This involves famishing yourself, both physically and emotionally, to an extent that when you finally get down to eat there's no stopping you. This can result in weight gain and developing eating disorders such as anorexia and binge eating.

When fasting intermittently, it can be quite tricky to identify and fulfil your body's nutritional needs since one has to ignore their hunger cues for as long as the fasting period lasts. This can have a direct impact on your relationship with hunger which is why it is recommended that you consult a competent physician or nutritionist to determine your nutritional requirements during IF.

Besides, you can always extend your eating window to ensure that you have enough time to eat properly and give your body all the nutrition it needs to function effectively.

Dehydrating yourself

Most of us struggle to drink the recommended amount of water each day. But this problem can quickly exacerbate when one is fasting since any hydration we get from food sources is blocked out too.

Dehydration can cause lethargy, muscle weakness, headaches and dizziness. And these can highly affect a person when they're already fasting.

The solution is quite simple since IF does not restrict water intake. You can drink water during and after the fasting period or enjoy a cup of black tea or coffee, depending on your mood. Some people also suggest drinking bone or veggie broth during fasting but keep in mind that these may put brakes on autophagy and put you out of the fasted state.

If you're thinking diet sodas then let me clarify that they are a no-no. But you can drink sparkling water to make yourself feel fuller when initially locking yourself into long fasts.

Even though the above mistakes are quite common, they aren't difficult to fix. Which means it isn't the end of the world even if you've found yourself doing some of these.

And while the above discussion can help you mend the mistakes and make the most of your IF regimen, it may raise some valid questions and concerns in your mind. You might find yourself wondering if something you're currently doing is right or if there is a recommended approach with regard to a certain aspect of IF. Therefore, the next chapter is dedicated to answering some of your more common and frequently asked questions about practicing IF.

Stay tuned!

Ch 8: Merry Questions & Answers

What you've been asking most frequently

This chapter tackles your most frequently asked questions (FAQs) and concerns regarding IF to help clear up your mind about the practice. Hope you find something valuable in here!

"I used to think I knew all the answers. Then I thought I knew maybe a few of the answers. Now I'm not even sure I understand the questions. Nobody knows anything."

— Pete Nelson, I Thought You Were Dead

Yes. We are usually far less aware than we care to think.

But it is also said that you can seek awareness if you ask the right questions. And previously, I did not know what that meant. That was until I performed a simple Google search and it all dawned upon me.

I had just found out that I was pregnant and that my partner was leaving me because he didn't want a child. This news initially had me numbed but as I regained consciousness, it felt as if the walls around me were caving in. My anxiety went through the roof and I started having the worst panic attacks within a matter of days. In a desperate attempt to salvage my sanity and improve my deteriorating situation, I began looking into meditation since a family acquaintance told me it had helped them a lot.

Owing to a lack of funds to engage a professional meditation teacher, I was forced to resort to dear old Google for guidance. However, as I was searching for a particular type of meditation technique (transcendental meditation, to be exact), I came across a few drawbacks of the said method. This intrigued me to dig deeper and as the search results for my latest Google query loaded in front of my eyes, it struck me...

Whatever results Google comes up with depend on what you type in the search bar. In my case, for instance, typing 'transcendental meditation techniques' yielded a bunch of top techniques for the practice while typing-in 'transcendental meditation disadvantages' scoured the internet for the disadvantages only. While this isn't some ground breaking information nobody never knew before, it taught me an important lesson:

You always get the answers you're looking for!

The above is true for everything and highlights the importance of asking the right questions to get the most valuable answers for yourself.

When it comes to IF, people usually have a lot going on in their minds. A vast majority is just entering the world of IF and is fascinated by all the information available on the subject. In fact, there is so much information accessible online that sometimes it becomes difficult to focus on the most important facts and to make important decisions based on them. This information overload usually gives way to analysis-paralysis and people find it easier to just give up.

Besides, some folks don't know much about the practice to begin with, and therefore couldn't answer the right questions.

And as we now know, asking the right questions is paramount to getting all the right answers.

Which is why this chapter focuses on addressing some of the most common and relevant concerns on the subject of IF and answers the right questions for anyone interested in the practice.

Disclaimer: While you may find that some of these questions have been tackled in the previous chapters, I've nonetheless given a brief rundown of the answers in order to help refresh your memory and to keep those who might have skipped some earlier sections in the loop.

So what are we waiting for? Let's get into this!

Question

I just finished my last meal at 8pm and am aiming for a 16-hour fast. When calculating my fasting window, do I start counting from when I finished the meal or when I first started having it?

Answer

Technically, the fasting period begins when you've finished eating. Therefore, you should start counting your fasting hours as soon as you finished the last meal i.e. from 8pm onwards.

Question

What is the best time for the 8-hour eating window in the 16:8 method of IF?

Answer

As answered by a later question as well, it is best to schedule your eating window earlier in the day when your insulin sensitivity is relatively higher. This is because insulin sensitivity declines as the day progresses.

Also, you should try and schedule as much of your eating in the daytime as possible and avoid night time munching because eating at night produces a higher insulin response than otherwise. Prolonged night time eating can, therefore, lead up to lowered insulin sensitivity or type 2 diabetes and even make you gain excess weight.

Question

I can't live without my morning coffee, can I have it while still fasting?

Answer

You can have black coffee, tea, and water throughout your fasting period without having to worry about breaking your fast. In fact, anything under 50 calories does not presumably break your fast so it should be okay to have your coffee or tea with a hint of milk or cream in the mornings. (No more than a hint though! Don't break the fast!)

Remember that it is generally a good idea to keep yourself hydrated during fasting to prevent some of the side effects of the practice and also to numb those hunger pangs.

Question

I've heard all my life that breakfast was the most important meal of the day. Will skipping it have a negative effect on my health?

Answer

You're not alone in thinking this. As long as we can remember, breakfast has been touted as the most crucial meal of the day. However, in order to get to the bottom of your question, one has to assess whether it is indeed a healthy start to the day or just a marketing gimmick printing money for big corporations selling sugary cereals to the whole nation.

For starters, breakfast literally means breaking fast. You can do that in the morning or at noon, whenever you fancy. For instance, you're still having breakfast when fasting intermittently and having your first meal of the day at noon.

Secondly, even if you break your fast in the morning, there is nothing wrong with it as long as you take it as an opportunity to eat something healthy instead of the customary sugar-laden cereals, doughnuts, croissants and fruit juices.

Our usual breakfast model is meant to spike insulin levels first thing in the morning and thereby reduce insulin sensitivity throughout the day. In contrast to a healthy meal filled with protein and complex carbs (think bacon, eggs and whole-grain bread), the sugar bombs we consume in the name of breakfast do nothing but harm our bodies and are better skipped.

Therefore, if you find yourself eating nothing but healthy foods in the morning then by all means go ahead and indulge yourself so long as you're keeping track of your calorie intake.

Question

What should I eat when I'm not fasting?

Answer

Before I answer this one, I want you to understand that although IF doesn't put any restrictions on WHAT you should eat, you must still be mindful of your diet in order to maintain your overall health and let IF do the work you intended it to do.

With that being said, what you put in your mouth when you aren't fasting does not vary much from what is normally considered healthy. So try to include as much of the following foods as possible in your diet to make the most of IF and enjoy good health:

- Fresh fruits and veggies
- Whole grains
- Foods rich in proteins such as poultry, meat and fish
- Dairy
- Nuts, beans and seeds

And finally, don't forget to drink enough water!

Question

Which type of IF regimen should I follow?

Answer

The type of IF method which might be most suitable for you depends on a number of factors such as your lifestyle, the state of your health and your goals regarding the practice. It is also determined by how far along you are in your IF journey. While a beginner who's just dipping their toes into IF might benefit from the 16:8 method, a pro who is thinking about switching to an advanced level of IF might want to take a different route.

Question

What should I eat during the eating window?

Answer

Whatever you do, you should aim to eat a healthy, balanced and nutrient-dense diet during the eating windows in order to meet your body's nutritional needs.

Question

What is highly recommended, eating earlier in the day or later?

Answer

When fasting intermittently, it's just as important to time your meals correctly as deciding what to eat. Although the practice itself doesn't dictate anything about the timing nor the types of food to consume, it is in your own best interest to give these some thought so you can make the most of your IF regimen and maintain a good overall health.

Research suggests that insulin sensitivity is the highest earlier in the day and declines as the day progresses. This implies that you should aim to time your eating window such that most of your food consumption happens in the early hours of the day and that you avoid nighttime (particularly late night) munching as much as is possible.

Food that is devoured late after sundown also has the effect of generating a greater insulin response than that consumed during daytime. If you stick to this eating pattern for long periods of time, you can risk decreasing your insulin sensitivity which can lead to type 2 diabetes.

Therefore, try to maintain an IF schedule that will allow you to consume all your major meals while the day is still somewhat young and quit eating as soon as you can in the evenings, if possible.

Question

Will my circadian rhythms be affected by IF?

Answer

Studies conducted on rodents show that IF can have a positive impact on circadian rhythms depending on the feeding times (eating windows). In this context, IF is considered a strong metabolic cue to regulate circadian rhythms. In simple terms, depending on how you've set your eating window, IF can have a positive impact on regulating your circadian rhythms.

Question

How hard it is to break and then resume an IF regimen?

Answer

Now this is an interesting question.

The difficulties you'll face as a result of breaking and then resuming an IF regimen depend on how long you've been practicing IF and the length of the break you took from the practice.

If you're, say, just three weeks into IF and took a week-long break then it should be relatively easy to make a comeback.

These 7 days of break from abstinence won't do much harm even if you've been fasting intermittently for as long as 8 months. However, you might find yourself in some serious trouble if this break extended to a month in which case it is recommended that you take your time to get back on track.

The main issue with prolonged breaks is that your carbs and sugar levels tend to elevate as you start eating normally which makes it harder to fast for longer periods of time. When trying to get back in the groove of things it is, therefore, recommended that you cut back on sugar and carbs first and rely more on proteins and healthy fats. With time, you'll find it much easier to continue with the IF regimen you used to follow.

Question

Will I lose muscle as a result of fasting intermittently?

Answer

If you could recall, the typical hierarchy for breakdown of nutrients for energy is as follows (starting from the highest priority to the lowest):

1. Carbs
2. Fat
3. Protein

Since protein is usually broken down as a last resort for providing fuel for the body, losing muscle shouldn't be a concern while fasting intermittently. Additionally, while IF allows you to abstain from food long enough that your body starts burning fat (aka ketosis), it doesn't deprive it to the extent that the muscle mass needs to be broken down for energy.

However, if you're a person who does some form of high-intensity interval training then it's a different story. Intense workouts in a fasted state may lead to the breakdown of muscle mass along with depleting fat reserves in the body. A solution is to treat yourself with a pre-workout snack high in carbs so that your muscles can be spared when the body needs more energy during an intense workout session.

Question

How to ensure that I eat enough during IF when weight loss isn't one of my goals?

Answer

Even if you aren't fasting intermittently for the sole purpose of losing weight, you must ensure that you're eating enough nutrient-dense food to meet your body's nutritional needs. This is particularly relevant during IF when your eating windows are limited and you have to make all your food choices during a fixed time period.

One way to make sure that you're eating enough nutritional foods is to plan ahead of time so you know what you'll be dining on, say, each day of the upcoming week. Another approach you can take in this regard is to maintain a food journal which tracks what you're eating when you aren't fasting. This is an effective form of mindful eating which can easily help you track what you're eating in a day and whether you've eaten enough to meet your daily nutritional needs.

Question

Can I exercise while fasting?

Answer

Working out when you're fasting is completely normal and doable, so long as you know what you're doing.

And by that I mean that you have to be mindful of a few things before you put on your trainers and head to the gym.

First and foremost, whether or not you will be able to exercise in a fasted state depends on the type of training/exercise you normally do. High intensity training is usually more difficult to accomplish while fasting than normal exercise.

Secondly, in order to be able to gain the maximum benefit from your workout regimen when fasting, you have to listen closely to your body. Don't expect yourself to ace that cardio routine when your body screams for a break and calls for refueling.

Besides, timing your meals is of utmost importance when working out during IF. Unless you're doing light exercises for general health purposes (in which case the timing of breaking your fast isn't that important), high intensity training requires that you fuel yourself up properly in order to have ample energy for your training and to prevent muscle breakdown.

One solution is to do 'Carb Cycling' which involves consuming more carbohydrates on days that you train while devouring more protein and fat when you don't.

Whatever you do, training while fasting intermittently requires a bit of experimentation to see what works for you. Still, it is recommended that you don't uproot your current workout routine and try to manage your IF regimen around what you currently have going.

Question

How do I match my training to my fasting schedule?

Answer

Matching your training with your fasting schedule can be extremely important, particularly when you're involved in high-intensity training that aims to increase athletic performance.

You can train both within a fasted or fed state, depending on how well your body copes with it and the intensity of your training. What's important is to listen to your body and adjust accordingly. Consider your most preferable time and intensity for training and adjust your fasting window appropriately.

For example, if you're due for a cardio session, adjust your 16:8 fast such that you eat a high-carb meal right before the training or consume a nutrient-dense healthy grub as soon as you're done.

Whatever you do, listen closely to how you feel and don't push yourself too hard.

Question

Can I drink diet soda and calorie-free energy drinks while fasting?

Answer

There is some controversial opinion on this one.

While some say that drinking diet soda and calorie-free energy drinks won't break your fast since these are technically 'calorie-free', others advocate against it.

This is because these otherwise calorie-free drinks contain artificial sweeteners such as 'Aspartame' which can trigger an insulin response in the body. Remember, we're trying to trigger ketosis and an insulin response won't help with that.

Question

Can I take supplements when I fast?

Answer

Supplements are an important part of your diet that must be taken regularly after consulting with your physician.

Fasting doesn't mean that you should stop taking supplements. However, there are certain supplements that can be taken during a fast without the risk of breaking it. For details on the supplements that can be taken during fasting, refer to the list below;

Supplements that don't break your fast:

- Multivitamins- those without added sugars and fillers
- Creatine
- Collagen- may slightly impact autophagy
- Probiotics and prebiotics
- Individual supplements for certain nutrients such as Vitamin A & D, zinc and copper- some of these are best taken with a meal though!
- Fish (or algae) oil- contains few calories

Question

Weight loss isn't my goal. Why should I fast intermittently then?

Answer

IF has more benefits than just weight loss. If you find that you don't need to shed excess pounds, you can still do IF to reduce the risk of type 2 diabetes, improve cardiovascular health, minimize the risk of cancers, decrease inflammation and reap some benefits for your mental health such as increased focus and alertness.

Besides, IF can also yield some benefits for your personal life as well such as simplifying your routine and saving time and money by reducing the amount of meals you consume in a day.

Question

How should I prepare myself to fast intermittently?

Answer

Preparing yourself before fasting intermittently can go a long way to ensure that you achieve your goals with the practice. This preparation must be done both mentally and physically and will typically involve the following;

Mental preparation:

- Consult your physician about any health conditions you may currently or potentially have
- Get clear on what you want to achieve with IF. Is it weight loss, lower inflammation or an overall good health?
- Choose how you'll do it. You may prefer the 16:8 method as a beginner or consider taking the 5:2 route. Don't be too hard on yourself in the beginning
- Get prepared for the side effects which may be more severe early on in the practice

Physical preparation:

- Identify your calorie needs to ensure that you get the most out of your IF regimen
- Reduce the intake of addictive substances such as alcohol and nicotine well before you begin IF to make it easy on yourself when you do fast
- Start making small yet healthy changes to your diet beforehand so your body has to work a little less hard while fasting. For instance, cut back on sugars and processed foods. This will also help make fasting relatively easier for you
- Since IF will considerably reduce the types of liquids you can consume, drink a lot of healthy fluids in the pre-fasting period to prevent dehydrating yourself
- Do light exercises to increase blood circulation and lymphatic drainage and plan to get plenty of rest so you don't overwhelm yourself

Question

Why do I get headaches during IF and how to avoid them?

Answer

Headaches are a common occurrence, along with weakness, nausea and irritability, especially when you're just starting on an IF regimen. Fasting triggers headaches mainly due to low blood sugar levels since you aren't consuming any calories in the fasted state. Additionally, an increase in the levels of stress hormone cortisol may also bring on a throbbing headache during fasting.

While fasting-induced headaches can resolve on their own as a person gets used to the regimen, there are certain things you can do to help with these before they raise their nasty heads and spoil your whole day:

- Eat less carbs during the eating window and rely more on fats and proteins to avoid the rapid blood sugar fluctuation associated with consuming carbs
- Keep yourself adequately hydrated to avoid headaches brought on by dehydration
- Try to monitor and reduce your caffeine intake in the pre-fasting period to avoid headaches associated with caffeine withdrawal
- Do your best to steer clear of the general triggers of headache such as stress, lack of sleep and fatigue
- If you find headaches a common occurrence, consider taking preventive medication (ones whose effects will last for the majority of the fasting period) before fasting to avoid having to deal with a terrible headache in the first place

Question

Am I starving myself as a result of IF?

Answer

Before I take this one on, I want you to understand the concept of starvation.

Starvation mode (or more technically, adaptive thermogenesis) is a natural response which is triggered when there is a long term deficiency of calories. This process kicks off by reducing the consumption of calories on hand, making a person feel hungrier and stimulating food cravings. It is also marked with the body preserving its fat reserves and utilizing muscle mass (protein) for energy instead.

However, the starvation protocol isn't initiated by short term fasting (aka IF). in fact, its just the conversational usage of the term 'starvation' that has us thinking that we'll starve as a result of IF when technically nobody starves in the modern world.

Therefore, to think that you'll starve yourself as a result of IF and have muscle breakdown is a wrong notion unless you're fasting totally for days at length, which is neither practical nor recommended.

Question

Is IF safe for women?

Answer

While it can't be distinctly concluded if IF is safe for women or not, this much is certain; IF may yield different results for men and women. And in the absence of conclusive evidence and in-depth research, it can be reasonably assumed that more women than men may find out that they may take more time to find a working model and get used to intermittent fasting.

The general guidelines on IF for women prescribe that pregnant or breastfeeding women should be wary of attempting to fast intermittently unless closely supervised by a healthcare professional. This is because these women require more calories in general and IF would inhibit that significantly.

Besides, if you're a stay-at-home or working pregnant mom, you already have a lot of claims on your limited energy reserves which is why IF may not be the ideal route for you.

Some women also report irregularities in their menstrual cycles and an early onset of menopause as a result of fasting intermittently. This can be attributed to the fact that the body of a female is highly sensitive to calorie intake which can directly affect some key functions related to hormone regulation. A disruption in these hormones, particularly those associated with reproduction, may ultimately lead to an erratic menstrual cycle, poor bone health and even infertility.

Owing to these factors, women are suggested to go for a modified IF approach which comprises of shorter fasting periods and fewer fasting days. Moreover, fasting under the supervision of a physician can be invaluable in this regard. This is because an experienced health professional can point you in the right direction when things don't seem right and might help you devise a suitable IF plan for yourself.

There is also something called Doctor Body too as well, which is basically listening in closely to what your body tells you as you practice IF. Negative symptoms like those mentioned above are signs that your body is undergoing change when we bring lifestyle alterations in the form of intermittent fasting to it. The key is to track them and see what happens in the longer while. If you have been practicing IF for two to four months, and the symptoms persist throughout, then seeking a physician for further advice could be crucial in determining why IF isn't working for you. However, if Doctor Body actually rebalances itself out and you emerge in a far better state of health, then those earlier negative symptoms were just symptoms of change, and that your body was able to sort itself out through your practice of IF. This does not mean I do not endorse seeking medical help, but rather it is more of asking for that bit of time to allow the body to adjust.

Question

How to fast intermittently when I'm on vacation?

Answer

IF should not come in the way of enjoying some down time and vacationing. In fact, people swear by the effectiveness of IF as a tool for keeping their health on track when travelling to a different corner of the world starts to disrupt their eating and exercise routine.

However, if you think that sticking to your IF regimen as a globe trotter would be a child's play, I recommend that you think about that again.

All the same, here are some tips to ensure that your IF regimen remains intact (as much as is possible) while you're out and about having the time of your life:

- Adjust the fasting period so you can make the most out of your vacation without putting your IF regimen in jeopardy. For instance, if you follow the 16:8 method of IF, you can try and move back your dinner an hour earlier and enjoy breakfast sooner the next day. You might even have to move your fasting time around more than once and that is completely okay if this lets you enjoy those precious moments with your loved ones while working on your health simultaneously. Most importantly, remember to go with the flow and live in the moment and you should be good.

- Don't over complicate your life by trying to figure out when to eat during long flights that take you across multiple time zones. Because, let's be honest, you'll give up after a while.

Consider this. You just boarded a plane that is supposed to take you to another continent with a different timezone. The flight crew serves the food as scheduled and before you could delve into that seemingly delicious pasta, a thought stops you in your tracks, 'Is it the eating time yet?'.

To figure out the answer to this daunting question, you summon all your mental math muscle and try to determine if your eating window has arrived. However, computing which timezone you're currently in and how much time has elapsed since your fasting window began makes your head spin. And here's what you finally decide; whatever, I'm going to give myself some well-deserved benefit of doubt and eat that pasta!

And that's perfectly fine. When finding yourself in a complicated situation like above, it is better to take a short break from IF and pick up where you left off upon reaching and settling in your destination. If you resist, chances are that you'd be ravenous when the plane lands and then more prone to eating whatever comes your way in quantities that you may later regret.

Better safe than sorry, right?

- I understand that being on vacation means exploring and enjoying all the adventurous activities that you've been dying to do. However, if you don't want to mess up your IF regimen while doing so, I have some pretty useful advice for you. Pour some thought into planning your adventures such that the most energy-intensive endeavors are tackled when you're in your eating window while you can still carry out all the low key activities in the fasted state. This will ensure that you don't overwhelm yourself while fasting by going mountain hiking when you're already low on energy.

- Plan for your macros thoughtfully. Travel exposes you to a variety of native cuisines that might not entail what you're used to at home. Therefore, you must try and keep track of what you're consuming in order to ensure that you're eating enough macronutrients while fasting intermittently.

  For instance, this one time I went to Europe for a small vacation with a group of friends. All we could find to eat in a small town in Western Europe was pizza, croissants, pasta and bread (along with some seriously next-level wine!). Before long, I was craving for some protein and had to scour the neighborhood for a small restaurant that served steaks. When the waiter finally put that perfectly cooked platter of medium-rare beef in front of me, I swear I could have cried some very happy tears!

  My advice? Try to switch between the offerings of the local cuisine to ensure you're getting all of your macros (particularly protein). This will ensure that you remain full for longer and help avoid those eerie blood-sugar fluctuations associated with consuming a diet laden with carbs.

- Be prepared for some adjustments when you're finally back from your wanderings. This is because no matter how hard you try to carry on with your IF regimen while travelling, you'll need to improvise for when you reach the comfort of your own home again.

  Travelling, particularly for longer periods of time, can make your biological clock go awry and it will take some time for it to get back on track. Give your body a moment to get in the groove of things and slowly work your way back towards the IF routine you used to follow. Meanwhile, rely on shorter fasting periods and fewer fasting days to train your body back to your desired IF regimen.

- Give yourself a break.

  And yeah, I know you're travelling and thereby already have some plans in place for indulging yourself. But consider taking a break from IF itself or at least limit fasting to an extent that won't interfere with your travel itinerary. This won't make the earth spin a little faster or your email load a bit slower!

  Life will go on even if you skip IF for a bit. So why not enjoy that trip to the Bahamas that you've been planning for years without worrying about the eating and fasting windows?

And finally, keep yourself hydrated, drink plenty of water, black coffee and tea and keep tabs on how much sleep you're getting to make the most of your IF regimen while you're on the go. Remember, IF is a flexible regimen that can be adapted to where you are in life and travelling does not have to be an exception to that!

Question

How to manage my social commitments while fasting intermittently?

Answer

In my opinion, managing your social commitments while fasting intermittently is easier than when you're following a strict diet plan that won't allow any wiggle room whatsoever.

This question also makes me remember a story that involves a dear friend of mine.

Let me introduce you to Katy, my friend, who had always been the most health-conscious of the lot. Katy had just started the keto diet and would stay away from pasta, rice and other high-carb foods like the plague.

So here's what a typical night out with her looked like.

Every. Single. Time.

The first step (as always) would be to pick the fanciest place that we could afford to eat at. Then, as the rest of us scrolled through the menu trying to pronounce some lavish Italian dish and making a fool of ourselves, Katy would become all restless. A few dozen atrociously funny jokes later and after hurtling a bunch of humorous insults all around, nearly everyone would start placing their orders.

Except Katy.

Who is now the only one who still has yet to decide. As we all waited for her to say something, she would reluctantly order a salad or side for the lack of a better option. The worst part is that, more often than not, that salad or side would taste like shit!

But hell! Katy had a diet to follow after all.

Thankfully, IF can save you the awkwardness my dear friend had to deal with AND some horrible food that many restaurants have to offer in the name of keto or some other fancy diet. For starters, you don't have to follow a strict diet plan that authoritatively dictates what you can and cannot have. Secondly, you can always adjust your IF schedule in accordance with your social commitments (consider having a late breakfast after a night out with your amigos) or just skip your regimen for a day and come back to it later.

That is precisely the beauty of a flexible regimen such as IF.

You can be healthy AND happy.

Not much in this world offers both!

Question

Is IF a long term solution for weight loss?

Answer

In order to determine if IF is a long term solution for weight loss, it helps to understand how it actually works to make a person shed excess pounds to begin with.

IF promotes weight loss by allowing an individual to consume fewer calories (hopefully). It works because when a person has to wait for the eating window in order to put even a single morsel of food inside their mouth, they automatically consume fewer calories than they normally would. This is, of course, assuming that they don't eat like its the end of the world when they've finally hit the eating hours.

Besides, IF also helps a person become leaner by optimizing some hormones related to controlling weight. One of these hormones is insulin. As insulin levels drop when a person fasts, the fat reserves in the body are activated to produce the much-needed energy. In contrast, the insulin levels aren't lowered if a person keeps eating normally in our present age, prompting their fat reserves to remain idle and thereby intact.

A short term fasting regimen akin to IF is also shown to increase metabolism, which can support weight loss. But can IF be considered a long term solution for weight loss? That really depends on a few things.

Whether IF can be expected to work in favor of weight loss in the long haul depends on how you approach the practice. People who have experienced some long term weight loss benefits from the regimen proclaim that they eat healthy outside the fasting window and incorporate some form of exercise in their daily routine to maintain the lost pounds. They also warn that once a person goes back to their normal eating patterns and discontinues IF, they can reasonably expect to gain their lost weight back and perhaps even more!

Besides, many people practicing IF find that it is quite sustainable. This implies that, when approached properly, the associated weight loss benefits of the practice can also be expected to stick around.

Remember, IF is more of a lifestyle change than a diet. If you're able to incorporate it successfully into your daily routine and see some positive results, then chances are that you'll stick to it for good. However, any benefits of the practice in the long term (including weight loss) will only transpire if you approach it with the right mindset and reasonable expectations.

Question

Can IF prevent aging and diabetes?

Answer

Let's begin by talking about the effects of IF on diabetes prevention. Whether or not IF can help prevent diabetes remains a topic of debate, and in the absence of any conclusive evidence, I would suggest taking any information available on the subject with a grain of salt.

Here's why.

IF is better than traditional fasting in that it allows for an eating window in between fasting periods, therefore being relatively safer for people with diabetes. With that being said, it still isn't considered a mainstream treatment for diabetes so indulging in it comes with its own risks.

What we do understand is that IF helps our body manage its blood sugar levels effectively and might help increase insulin sensitivity. It also gives the liver and pancreas, two main organs involved in managing glucose and producing insulin, a well-deserved break from their usual tasks.

But studies conducted on the role of IF in preventing or controlling diabetes are extremely small in scope to be considered conclusive. Additionally, much of the research on the subject has been conducted on lab animals, which needs to be extended to include a lot more humans if we are to extract some reliable and relevant results from these.

To sum it up, IF can be effective in preventing diabetes or even treating pre-diabetes. However, if you're someone who has diabetes and is looking at IF as a solution to your health problems, you need to understand all the risks involved and must not begin fasting intermittently without first consulting your physician. I'd put it out there that it is better to be safe than sorry when it comes to health. I know a number of reputable physicians out there who have published books touting that IF CAN cure diabetes, but again, due to the fact that clinical trials done on people aren't of a sufficient number, the consensus out there is still to approach this particular issue with some care. Personally though, I would vouch for its veracity. Purely because I have got anecdotal evidence! 10 of my friends and family who are diabetic or pre-diabetic did the IF lifestyle change and saw their health status improve. 10 out of 10. Sounds good enough to me!

Now let's explore the second part of the question i.e. if IF can prevent aging?

I'll be honest. When I was doing my research on IF, the anti-aging benefits of the practice caught my attention the most. I mean, who doesn't want to lock in time and remain as young as possible for as long as possible?

I don't know about you, but count me in if there's anything like that involved. And I promise to never look back!

On a serious note, IF has been shown to have anti-aging effects.

As we age, things (such as metabolism) slow down while greying hair and wrinkles on the skin pick up the pace. Aging is a natural process and there is no denying that. However, a slower metabolism can cause a host of health issues such as weight gain.

A short term fasting regimen such as IF has shown to spur metabolism which makes the body burn calories more efficiently and keeps weight gain at bay (unless you're doing something else to contribute to putting on excessive weight). IF also reduces the degeneration of DNA, which is another facet of aging, while helping to repair damaged hereditary material at the same time. It triggers cell autophagy, thereby helping the body clear up damaged and dead cells and cell components (we discussed autophagy in a previous chapter) and also helps increase antioxidants in the body to prevent cell damage.

As the years pass on, the human body can also experience chronic inflammation and the loss of lean muscle mass. Inflammation, in particular, is also suspected to be caused by the modern eating patterns and diets we indulge in on a daily basis. IF can help in this regard by suppressing inflammation that not only occurs naturally but is also brought on by our poor eating habits. Besides, IF has been shown to cause a spike in Human Growth Hormone that can prevent the loss of lean muscle mass as we age and boost fat burning.

Even if IF can't be touted as the best anti-aging remedy that exists to date, considering all of these collective benefits of the practice, it can be reasonably stated that it can help a person enjoy a better quality of life for a relatively longer period of time.

And that, in itself, can be anti-aging for most of us!

Question

How often do I have to fast intermittently in order to experience weight loss?

Answer

As I have been reinforcing since the beginning of this book, IF is a flexible practice that can be adapted to suit your circumstances and lifestyle. Keeping that in mind, how often you fast intermittently depends on which IF method fancies you the most and works out for your style of living.

With that being said, weight loss technically occurs when you burn more calories than you consume, i.e. develop a calorie deficit. Therefore, whatever IF method pans out for you and helps you achieve a calorie deficit is the one to go for when talking about weight loss.

Depending on your daily routine and lifestyle, this can either be the 16:8 method or the 5:2 regimen. All you need to do is pick one and then stick to it for a certain period of time to see if you experience any positive results. If something doesn't work out, that's fine as well. Just switch to another method and see how that goes until you find the one that's perfect for you.

Question

How long does it take for IF to show the weight loss results?

Answer

IF works differently for everybody primarily because not everyone's metabolism works the same and each individual has their own personal preferences when it comes to the practice. Moreover, how fast it shows results when it comes to weight loss also depends on how you're eating outside the fasting window.

Some studies show that results typically become apparent over the 10-week mark while others demonstrate that weight loss occurs over a period of 3-12 or even 3-24 weeks. But before you take these numbers as conclusive, I must warn you that these studies vary considerably with respect to the number of participants or how much weight loss or body fat reduction IF was able to achieve in each case.

A good rule of thumb, however, is to give whatever IF regimen you're following a month or two to work before switching to another method and be mindful of anything you might be doing wrong that can mess with the results.

Question

What is the most effective IF regimen in terms of weight loss?

Answer

I'll answer this one based on a criteria that I had set for myself when I was just beginning IF and weight loss was my absolute number-one goal for the practice.

For me, the most effective IF regimen meant two things; something that gave me actual results that I could count on AND that naturally worked so well for me that I had no problem incorporating it into my daily routine (unlike some other regimens that made me flinch every time I so much as thought about them!).

Based on the criteria above and my own personal experience, I found out that the 16:8 method worked perfectly well for weight loss as I was just dipping my toes into the water with IF.

Not only is this method extremely user-friendly when you're just starting out, it also works on a simple yet basic and effective principle i.e. fasting for 10-16 hours prompts the body to go into ketosis mode and thereby burn fat.

With that being said, everybody has their personal preferences when it comes to which IF regimen to follow and the same IF method may yield different results for different people. This is why it is recommended that you experiment with these methods to figure out which of them yields the most impressive results for you while also being practical for your lifestyle.

Remember, the best way is always the way that works for you.

Question

IF vs Calorie Restriction-which is better for weight loss?

Answer

Glad you've asked!

According to research, none exceeds the other when it comes to weight loss and fat mass loss.

Research conducted on the effects of daily and intermittent Calorie Restriction on weight loss, fat mass loss and lean mass reduction in overweight and obese adults reveals that there are no significant differences between how the two approaches work as far as weight loss and fat mass loss is concerned. However, intermittent Calorie Restriction diets may be more effective for lean mass retention than daily Calorie Restriction diets.

You might ask then, what's the difference? Well, the difference arises depending on whether we're talking about long term weight loss or short term.

And Dr. Jason Fung, author of The Obesity Code, explains it in much detail.

According to him, the main difference between daily Calorie Restriction diets (DCR) and IF can be explained by the metabolic slowdown brought about by DCR diets. And to understand this, we have to go a little deeper into how our bodies work.

Dr. Fung explains this phenomenon by referring to an American reality TV show called 'The Biggest Loser'. The show involves participants, who have struggled with weight issues their entire lives, compete to lose the most weight through some tough physical, mental and emotional challenges. Whoever exhibits the strongest nerves while losing the most weight at the same time becomes the winner and banks in on a hefty $100,000 prize.

The show is meant to change how the participants eat, move and think and offers them a chance to change their lifestyles in favor of a healthier one.

Not so much in reality!

And to explain just why, Dr. Fung quotes a former contestant of the show stating that a reunion never happens because "We're all fat again". Thanks to a phenomenon known as 'Metabolic Slowdown' which is a well-known side effect of DCR diets.

Here's how it happens.

As we decrease our daily intake of calories, our Resting Metabolism Rate (the energy required to sustain our basic bodily functions such as breathing and heartbeat) slows down in response to the lower energy available. As soon as the calorie expenditure goes below calorie intake owing to the slower RMR, the weight gain resumes. If you remember, this is everything going against the calorie deficit principle which involves a higher calorie expenditure as compared to consumption.

And maintaining this calorie deficit is primarily the reason a person loses weight and maintains it.

However, when the opposite happens in response to the DCR diets, you just can't expect the same results. Granted, there is weight loss in the beginning. But a person stops losing weight in the long haul and even begins putting it on back again due to lower RMR as described above.

You might also remember that we talked about how IF does NOT put our bodies in starvation mode since shorter periods of fasting do not initiate the same protocols as required by starvation. Well, DCR diets have been found to have the opposite effect. These tend to put your body in starvation mode and as soon as you try to come out of it by increasing your calorie intake, the lost pounds come running back like your worst nightmare.

Dr. Fung explains that long-term weight loss is only possible if you somehow maintain your RMR or Basal Metabolism Rate, as it is also known. He highlights a very important paradox; what doesn't put a person in starvation mode is a form of (controlled) starvation itself, aka IF.

While the short term weight loss effects of CR diets and IF are more or less the same, the outlook is drastically different when things are looked at in the longer term. The CR diets put a person on starvation mode by lowering their BMR, precisely what the IF prevents, and thereby do not aid in losing and maintaining weight loss in the long term.

Question

How long does it take to get used to IF?

Answer

Nutrition experts recommend that you must give your body at least 5 days to get used to a new eating pattern. With that being said, the time it takes for a person to become accustomed to IF depends on a number of factors such as:

- Diet: if you're used to eating a high-carb diet then you might be in for some trouble. This is because the glucose obtained from breaking down carbs causes rapid blood sugar fluctuations. As soon as your blood sugar drops during fasting, you'll start getting hunger signals (and strong ones at that!) which can be quite difficult to ignore.

  On the contrary, if you favor a diet high in protein and fat while consuming carbs only in moderation, you stand a better chance of fasting without much difficulty. This is because protein and fat have the tendency to keep you full for a longer time therefore downplaying the hunger pangs and allowing you to survive the fasting period with much more success.

- Hydration; One is also more likely to struggle with fasting if they aren't well hydrated. Drinking water and fluids not only help flush out the toxins produced through fasting but are a great source of nutrients such as sodium, potassium and magnesium to help you get through abstinence intact.

Dehydration can result in fatigue, headaches and a dry mouth, all of which can make fasting more challenging than it needs to be.

- Trying to do too much too soon; IF enthusiasts that are just starting off can sometimes go over the board and think they can pull off longer fasts without much problem. But just like any other regimen, the body needs to get used to shorter periods of fasting before it can transition to longer and more challenging fasts.

  If, on top of having an aggressive fasting schedule, you have zero experience with fasting then things can be more grim for you. The trick is to take it slow and give yourself enough time to get used to the practice.

  Slow and steady wins the race. Remember?

Question

How to fight with mental fog or fatigue during IF?

Answer

While some people claim that IF brings greater mental clarity and focus for them, there are others who find it hard to concentrate when they're fasting. The latter may be beginners or those who are transitioning to a more advanced IF regimen. Whatever the case, experiencing mental fog and fatigue can be pretty normal when you're fasting and can be dealt with through one or more of the following ways:

- Staying hydrated. Drinking plenty of water and other fluids during fasting as well as the eating window can prevent you from feeling fatigued and washed out

- If a lack of caffeine is the cause of your decreased cognitive function, try some black coffee or tea (unsweetened) to invigorate yourself. Such calorie-free beverages will not only give you the boost you need but also won't put a dent in your fast. Talk about win-wins!

- Hop onto the yoga mat and try some mindfulness techniques such as meditation or a set of yoga stretches aimed at increasing focus. I can guarantee that you'll feel better afterwards.

- If yoga and meditation isn't your thing, try some simple but lightweight physical exercises to get yourself in the groove of things. Doing a little bit of physical activity such as jumping jacks or squats allows your muscles to release that stored glycogen (aka glucose) and spikes up the blood sugar levels. Although not a very long term solution, this can charge you up for a short while at least

- When you're experiencing brain fog and fatigue and have just started IF, it might help to get some extra sleep until your body learns to cope with a lower calorie supply during fasting

- Time your eating windows such that you can consume the most calories when you need to be the most alert. For example, if you tend to do more mental work earlier in the day, try to have small snacks throughout that time or plan a nice fulfilling breakfast before you get down to work.

The good news about having to deal with mental fog and fatigue during IF is that it usually doesn't last that long. As soon as your body becomes accustomed to the fasting regimen you're following, you'll notice a decline in these distressing occurrences and might even realize that you've never felt this good before.

Ch 9: Oh Those Impt Tips And Tricks!

Welcome to your arsenal of hacks!

Although I knew all too well about the various health benefits of IF, I began with just one major goal in mind.

Weight loss.

Gaining excess weight til being classified as obese was never an issue that I faced in my life before. However, after I became pregnant and saw my mental health go down the drain in the wake of some very grim life circumstances, the numbers on the weight scale started climbing.

And they climbed fast (I gained almost 5 lbs per week!)

So when I finally discovered IF and started my 16:8 regimen, I was hoping to see some tangible results, more sooner than later.

Unfortunately, during the initial foray into IF I was hardly seeing any improvement that I would deem satisfactory. Granted, I knew that IF wasn't some miracle that would fix things up in a heartbeat.

However, I still knew it was high time that I saw some results that I could count on.

Which led me to discover one of the hacks I'll be talking about in this chapter. In fact, it will be the first IF hack that I'll be sharing with you since I have personally benefited from it.

But here's my point

As a novice IFer who has only been at it for a few weeks, it can sometimes be tricky to figure out what you're doing wrong or how to approach things in a way that would yield some A-OK results for your health.

Which is where the tips and hacks we're about to cover come in play.

Ready to bolster up your arsenal with some really handy yet effective tips that might remove the only thing coming in the way of your success?

Let's dive in!

Hack #1- Use your hands to portion food

Now this is a very interesting hack and one of the first few that helped me reclaim my confidence in IF.

Our hands are a handy tool to do a lot of stuff. But did you know that you can also portion control with them?

After failing to lose any noticeable weight with the initial period of fasting intermittently, I became certain that I was doing something wrong.

But what was it?!

This question kept haunting me until one day I learned about portion control with hands. While I am well-aware of portion control and its virtues for effectively regulating the amount of calories one consumes and thereby maintaining a healthy weight, I never thought it would be relevant to IF in any manner.

And all of that with such practical tools which are literally attached to our bodies? You must be kidding me!

Using your hands to portion control is easier than you might think.

And if you aren't seeing any visible results with your weight loss even after fasting intermittently for a pretty reasonable amount of time (think 10-12 weeks) then this may be what you're doing wrong!

Portion control with hands is a quick, convenient and fairly accurate method of measuring the portion sizes of protein, carbs and fats that you must consume in one sitting. This is because not only can you use this hack when you're dining outside the comfort of your home but the size of your hands is also proportional to your body size, making them an excellent tool to determine how much to eat to fulfill your body's needs. Keeping these relative proportions in mind, all you have to do is take one look at your food, the other at your hand and determine your portion.

So here's how this works. The next time you have a plate stacked high with some juicy chicken steak and roasted vegetables in front of you, here's exactly how to decide your cut for the day and leave the rest untouched (for another day and time, maybe).

- The palms of your hands determine your protein portions. This means that if you fully open and hold out your hand, the size of your palm indicates one serving size for meat.
- Your fists determine the portion of veggies that you must be consuming. The size of one of your clenched fists is equal to approximately one cup of those delicious vegetables that you must consume.

- Your cupped hands can be used as an indication for your carbs portion.
- The entire length of your thumb determines your fat portions.

In addition to the above,

- If you look at your thumb, from the top of your thumb to the knuckle is approximately one tablespoon.
- If you look at the tip of your index finger, that is approximately one teaspoon.
- If you look at the top of your clenched fist, that amounts to approximately ½ a cup.

If you remember, the underlying principles of weight loss dictate that you need to maintain a calorie deficit in order to lose weight effectively. This means that you must consume less calories than you spend.

Besides being extremely practical and easy, this hack will also help you keep track of your calorie intake so you can maintain a calorie deficit which is crucial for losing weight effectively. This can also be imperative to when you're trying to eat mindfully in your eating window instead of simply devouring whatever's in sight.

Hack #2- Time and money saving meal prep

We established this much in one of the earlier chapters; IF can save you both time and money by reducing the number of meals you have to prepare (and for a terribly slow-eater like me, eat!) as well as by cutting back on the food budget otherwise spent on snacks and other unhealthy foods.

Because, guess what, you probably won't be eating these anymore! (or eating waaay less of it at the very least)

With that being said, one might be left wondering about how to bank in on these time and $$$ saving benefits of IF in real life, particularly if they aren't familiar with meal-prepping to begin with. A common question in this regard might be:

How exactly to meal-prep in advance when I'm anticipating a busy week ahead and know for sure that there is a high risk of me ordering takeaway in a haste before the eating window closes?

You might also be contemplating if meal-prepping for an entire week ahead of time will turn out to be a task that is daunting beyond your reckoning or if it is simply practicable at all since food can go bad after a certain number of days?

In all honesty, I've got to say that you're probably overthinking a little and that meal-prepping isn't that frightening as you might think.

Particularly with the tips we're about to discuss.

The hacks included below are aimed at taking the guesswork out of any time and money saving meal preparation that might be underway for you and give some practical insights on what you could be doing instead of just speculating.

Or maybe even getting terrorized... (by the mere thought of meal planning!)

So brace yourselves and get ready to get your socks knocked off (and take some notes!)

- Many people find meal-prepping in advance frightening because of the amount of work involved in doing so. However, things don't seem so bad if you try and begin with preparing only for a few days at once.

  For instance, you can set aside two days of the week (say Sunday and Wednesday) for preparing some food in advance for the upcoming days. This will divide your work regarding meal-prepping for the entire week in two days instead of one, thereby making it less tiring and dreadful.

  As you become more adept at the practice, you can start preparing bigger batches and/or more meals within each session to cover up the entire week's meal-prepping in a single go.

  It gets easier with time, I promise.

- When you're just starting out, its usually a good idea to refrain from preparing overly complicated meals that need fancy ingredients. Instead, search and opt for simple meal-prep ideas and recipes that won't require much time and aren't only healthy but align well with how your taste buds feel.

A time-consuming recipe that involves a multitude of difficult-to-pronounce ingredients as well as needs to be prepared in countless steps might sound intriguing, but it is better to save it for days when you have more time on hand or want to feel a little more pampered than usual.

Whenever you can, stick with simple and easily-available ingredients and recipes that will allow you to whip up a meal in no time. Believe me, this goes a long way in ensuring that you don't get frustrated by the idea of meal-prepping in advance and prevent you from making bad food choices.

- Before I explain this next tip to you, a little disclaimer is in order;

  I understand that we're looking at ways to prep meals that will be as light on the budget as possible, but there are certain expenses that you have to undergo (consider these investments) in order to make all this meal-prepping thing work.

  For starters, think about spending some $$$ on pre-cut produce which isn't only convenient to use but will also save you the cost of eating out if cutting veggies and fruits is your pet-peeve.

  These pre-cut items of food are ready to use, whenever you are, and will save you enormous amounts of time that can be spent on other aspects of the meal-prepping mission such as making homemade sauces.

To make your life even easier, invest in some good quality knives for chopping up those fruits and veggies in the blink of an eye.

- Another meal-prep hack that might come in handy is to prepare big batches of homemade sauces and salad dressings, particularly if you aren't a big fan of the store-bought versions (due to obvious reasons).

  And while you're at it, consider storing your wet ingredients (such as salad dressings) separately from the dry ones (say, the vegetables for a veggie salad). This will ensure that your dry ingredients remain as crisp and fresh as possible.

  Besides, that satisfying feeling of pouring a delicious salad dressing over perfectly cut veggies is not to be taken lightly.

  At all!

- Cook your meat servings in a single batch. This is an amazing yet time saving hack that can spare you hours in the kitchen.

  Take all the protein that needs to be cooked/baked and divide it into small sections by making a few partitions in your baking tray with aluminum foil. Season each portion however you like and put it into the oven for a quick batch-bake.

In order to ensure that your batch turns out perfectly, cut all pieces of meat in roughly the equal size and put the same type of meat together in a single batch. This means that you must cook chicken with chicken and beef with beef since different meat types have varying cooking times.

When it comes to storing your meat, make sure to cut small pieces that are easier to reheat than larger chunks.

- Now this is another hack that will require some investment but will pay you off for years once you're done.

  Purchase a bunch of clear plastic (BPA free) or, better, glass containers for storing batches of food that you'll be preparing as part of your weekly meal prep. These clear containers will not only let you know about the contents inside instantly but also help you portion out your main course, sides and snacks.

  When shopping for your containers, keep certain factors such as being BPA free, food separation, size and air tightness in mind. Also, make sure that you factor in the size of these containers carefully so they can easily fix in your refrigerator/freezer, microwave and dishwasher.

- Consider freezing some stuff that can be used when the going gets really tough. While it is recommended that you refrigerate food for no more than a few days and freeze anything that needs to be stored for more than 4-5 days, it is generally a good idea to have some freezed food at hand for when you have a particularly crazy week or few days ahead.

Prepare some freezer-friendly foods such as pasta, soup and dumplings and try to store them in aluminum containers with lids. For ease of use, label these foods and reheat them when you are really stretched thin after a long day at work.

You will thank yourself for this one!

- Get that slow cooker up and running.

When was the last time you used your slow cooker to cook some food?

If your answer is couldn't remember? Me neither!

A slow cooker is the best set-it-and-forget-it tool you can get for your kitchen that will have some mouthwatering food ready for you and your family at the end of a long day. Unlike popular opinion, these can be used for brewing more than just stews. All you need to do is a little research on slow-cooker recipes and you might be pleasantly delighted.

Slow cooking not only brings out the flavour in your foods but is also a match made in heaven for foods that tend to stick to the bottom of pans and scorch or burn altogether.

They also allow you the opportunity to make bigger batches of your favorite foods which means you can store any excess if you're meal-prepping for the week ahead.

Just take that slow-cooker out of the storage (or buy one if you don't have any) and see how it transforms your life!

- If you're a smoothie-lover like me, you know how much trouble it is to get all the ingredients together before you can push that button on your food processor and enjoy a glass full of healthy smoothie.

  It almost takes all the fun out of it!

  But here's a solution. You can pre-package everything you need for that perfect smoothie into small plastic bags so that when it's time, all you need to do is empty the contents of the bag into the blender, push the right button and sip on the goodness you've just whipped up (or is blended the right word?).

  If you use milk or yogurt in your smoothies, you can also portion these beforehand in an ice-cube tray and then add whatever amount you need directly into the blender without having to fiddle with them at the last moment.

  What this has made me learn is this; small conveniences go a long way in improving our lives!

- Make room for leftovers by adding in a leftovers' night to your weekly plan.

  Leftovers are a reality, even if you've been the most diligent meal-planner on this planet.

  But throwing out food is not an ideal solution. Not only is it a waste of valuable resources but it also hurts our planet with food waste being one of the top contributors towards filling our landfills.

  But you don't really need to throw away food that wasn't consumed earlier (unless its gone bad, that's another story). What you can do, instead, is to plan a leftover night where you do nothing but warm up last night's pasta and call it a day.

  To spicc things up a bit and give it a more fresh feeling, you can stir fry some chicken and/or veggies in herbs and top the pasta off with them.

  And here you go. Dinner is served!

- Start prepping for your meal-prepping, as soon as you're back from the grocery store.

  Sorting and putting everything away when you've just returned from a long shopping spree at the grocery store can be extremely bothersome. You're all tired and exhausted from the long drive to and from the store as well as from walking around from one aisle to the other, looking for that coconut milk and refried beans that aren't where they used to be.

(Honestly, why do grocery stores do this? Is finding what you need among hundreds of aisles stacked high with products some new sport I haven't heard of?)

However, if you just stow away everything upon reaching home, you may find yourself in an even more annoying situation. And one that, unlike misplaced items in the grocery store, you can completely avoid.

So here's what you can do.

Wash and prep your herbs, portion out big chunks of meat as per your usage, rinse and pre-cut some of your veggies, take the eggs out of their cartons and put them in the egg tray in your refrigerator, slice your bread and put grains and nuts in air tight jars, to name a few.

Although daunting at first, these few additional steps will make your life a lot more easier when you're actually prepping your meals for the week ahead. Just take some of those pre-cut and rinsed veggies and throw an amazing salad together within minutes.

No fuss.

Who doesn't love that?

- Give a little love to your pantry and fridge. They'll return it many times over!

  Having an organized pantry and fridge can go a long way in helping you meal-prep effectively because you'll know what you have on hand as well as what you need. Additionally, a clean and well-maintained fridge and pantry allows you to get rid of stuff that you don't need (or won't ever use) to make room for things you can actually utilize to prepare healthy meals for yourself and your family.

  The next time you go grocery shopping, take a long look at your pantry and fridge before you leave to toss out anything that is useless or expired. Moreover, you must also try and store similar ingredients together for ease of use and put everything you'd use for that morning smoothie or evening bake in sight so you know when a backup is needed. You can also use some sticky notes to put manufacturing dates on your food containers (particularly for frozen items) and keep older food items in the front so they are used first.

  Some of these tips might sound like a no-brainer to you. But these little items really do stack up in helping out with kitchen productivity, so much so that when you actually slack off on doing this stuff that you realize its importance.

- Save yourself time, money and undue frustration by having a well-prepared grocery list on hand before you set foot outside the door of your house.

This may seem like another no-brainer (is there even a point to this list?!) but is actually something a lot of us do poorly or don't bother doing at all.

Having a well thought-out grocery shopping list will not only ensure that you don't miss out on anything but also might save you some money since you have a list of targeted items in mind and are less likely to deviate from it.

Back this up with a little research on what you want to prepare for the upcoming week, list down the precise ingredients that are required after taking stock of your pantry and fridge and nothing can come in your way of healthy eating.

All.Week.Long.

The above are just a few of the tips and hacks that you can use to make meal-prepping for a busy week easier. But if you're just starting out, the biggest advice I can give is to start small and build it up from there. For instance, begin by meal-prepping for one or two days of the week and then go on to prep food for the entire week once you find your rhythm.

Whatever it is that you do, these time and money saving meal-prep hacks will go far to ensure that you eat healthy and mindfully during your fasting window and make the most of your IF practice.

Hack #3- Nutrient dense food swaps

Nutrient dense food swaps are small yet intentional food switches that can have a big impact on your overall health.

They work on one fundamental principle; replacing unhealthy foods with real ones that actually have some nutritional value for our bodies.

Nutrient dense food swaps involve rethinking about what you've been consuming in the name of food (or worse, healthy food!) and switching it up with foods that are actually healthy for your body. This might seem a little difficult at first but is quite simple and doable once you get the hang of it.

Need some inspiration?

Included below is a list of food swaps that can come in handy when you find yourself in a food situation next time.

Food item

Potato chips and tortillas

What to swap 'em with!

Cruditès (sliced or whole raw vegetables)

Food item

Buns and sandwich bread

What to swap 'em with!

Sourdough bread or lettuce wraps

Food item

Regular fries

What to swap 'em with!

Baked sweet potato fries

Food item

White rice

What to swap 'em with!

Brown rice, quinoa, cauliflower rice or farro

Food item

Egg whites

What to swap 'em with!

Aquafaba (leftover liquid drained from canned chickpeas)

Food item

Egg

What to swap 'em with!

Chia seeds

Food item

Scrambled eggs

What to swap 'em with!

Tofu

Food item

Shredded meat

What to swap 'em with!

Jackfruit (add seasoning for taste)

Food item

Pasta

What to swap 'em with!

Spaghetti squash

Food item

Lasagna strips

What to swap 'em with!

Sliced zucchini

Food item

Brown sugar

What to swap 'em with!

Chopped fresh mangoes

Food item

Regular ice cream

What to swap 'em with!

Banana ice cream (non-processed)

Food item

Regular ground beef burger

What to swap 'em with!

Ground beef patty with 50% chopped mushrooms

Food item

Sour cream

What to swap 'em with!

Greek Yogurt or tahini

Food item

Mayonnaise

What to swap 'em with!

Mashed avocado or silken tofu

Food item

Soft Cheese

What to swap 'em with!

Cashew cream

Food item

Salt

What to swap 'em with!

Lemon zest and juice

Food item

Potato chips

What to swap 'em with!

In-shell pistachios

Food item

Sugary drinks

What to swap 'em with!

Water infused with fruit, unsweetened flavored tea or sparkling water

Food item

Pretzels

What to swap 'em with!

Macadamia nuts

Food item

Crackers

What to swap 'em with!

Bean snacks made from broad beans and chickpeas

Food item

Regular flour

What to swap 'em with!

Almond or green banana flour

Food item

White flour

What to swap 'em with!

Nut flour or pulses. Think black beans, peas and chickpeas

Food item

Regular pasta

What to swap 'em with!

Legume pasta

Food item

Oatmeal

What to swap 'em with!

High-fiber cereal

Food item

Processed deli meat

What to swap 'em with!

Sliced roasted chicken

Food item

Regular pizza topping

What to swap 'em with!

Topping with more veggies added in, like bellpeppers

Food item

Desserts

What to swap 'em with!

Naturally sweet fruit, like cherries or berries. Grapes too

Food item

Store bought jam

What to swap 'em with!

Mashed berries with lemon as a preservative or another homemade pure fruit spread

Food item

Frappuccino

What to swap 'em with!

Coffee with almond/coconut milk

Food item

Regular candy bars

What to swap 'em with!

Dark chocolate bars

Food item

Vegetable oil

What to swap 'em with!

Extra virgin olive oil

Food item

Processed fruit juice

What to swap 'em with!

Coconut water

Food item

Parmesan cheese

What to swap 'em with!

Nutritional yeast

Food item

Bottled salad dressings

What to swap 'em with!

Homemade dressings

Food item

Chocolate chips

What to swap 'em with!

Cacao nibs

Food item

Heavy cream

What to swap 'em with!

Cashew cream

Food item

Croutons

What to swap 'em with!

Pepitas

And the list goes on...

But you get the idea.

Nutrient dense food swaps are a great way to add nutrients to your diet. This is of paramount importance when you're fasting intermittently since you have to get all your macros and micros within a small eating window. Once that opportunity is gone, you're back to fasting and eating nothing, which itself becomes quite unsustainable if you aren't getting enough nutrition for your body while you can.

Hack #4- 5:2 minimal calorie day food choices

You might remember the 5:2 IF method where you eat like you normally would 5 days of the week, and limit your calorie intake (500 for men and 600 for women) for the rest of the week. While it is recommended that you don't overeat on the non-fasting days in order to lose weight effectively, a common question that gets asked is 'what should I eat on my calorie-restricted (fasting) days?'.

And that is a good question to ask since one must keep their calorie consumption on fasting days within bounds in order for the regimen to work, and because they have this restriction in place, ought to use their calorie budget wisely.

It's like you have one hour's worth of energy to do stuff and the choice to take your liberties with the chores that you prefer. What would you do?

Would you rather spend it idling around (or worse, thinking about what to do?) or use that limited energy to tackle the most pressing and important tasks on hand?

Its a similar choice you have to make when using the 5:2 method of IF since the calorie consumption on fasting days is quite limited. However, this does not mean that you have to slack on eating healthy and mindfully. Instead, it makes mindful eating even more important since you can't just spend your meager calorie budget thoughtlessly. Otherwise you risk facing consequences like dizziness, headaches, constipation, dehydration and the inability to cope with colder temperatures, to name a few.

Besides, a calorie restriction also does not mean that you have to starve. There are endless recipes and food choices you can look into that allow you to consume healthy and delicious food, all under your calorie budget.

The goal is to consume lower-calorie foods that are high in their nutritional value. Not to deny yourself completely while frantically counting calories.

For some motivation, here are a few food choices that'll work well with your 5:2 IF schedule without breaking your calorie bank. You can have them on their own or brew some delicious meals, the detailed recipes of which can be found anywhere on the internet, and enjoy a hearty luncheon even on the days you're fasting!

- Veggies. You can have as generous a portion as you like!
- Salads (make yourself an appetizing Asian chicken salad or go for a chicken and pineapple salad, equally good and both under 250 calories!)
- Low calorie cup soups
- Hard-boiled eggs
- Grilled or baked fish, chicken or lean meat
- Soups (think carrot and lentil soup or broccoli and kale green soup)
- Cauliflower rice bowls with chicken (approx. 400 calories)
- Black coffee, tea and sparkling water

The above list is not exhaustive. There exist a whole lot of other foods that you can consume during your fasting days, so long as you can keep a track of your calorie intake.

The aim of the above list is to provide some insight into the fact that you can eat healthy, scrumptious and filling meals even when you're fasting intermittently and are on a restrictive calorie budget for those two days.

Remember, fasting is not about starving yourself. One of the primary objectives of the practice is to help you make intentional decisions regarding your food so you can improve your overall health while losing excess weight.

Hack #5- Nip those cravings in the bud!

Dealing with food cravings can be tough, particularly when it is an especially chill night at home and you're in the mood for a good movie (or a book, whatever you fancy!)

But here's what's missing in that awesome plan of yours. SNACKS!

Really, is Netflix and that blockbuster movie ever complete without that ice-cold beer or a bag of your favorite potato chips?

But here's another dilemma. You're fasting intermittently and have to stop eating after 7pm. Which means that, technically speaking, you can't really have those potato chips.

Or that beer.

Or that pint of ice cream (if you're like me!)

Now I do understand that you can loosen up on your IF regimen every so often, but you can't always do that without a serious risk of putting all your efforts to waste.

So here's what to do in times like these (or when you're having a particularly lousy moment with IF and want to do something about it without having to screw your regimen forever)

- Fill yourself up with calorie-free beverages like unsweetened black coffee, tea or plain water. This will not only ensure that you don't get dehydrated during fasting but will also suppress your appetite, at least for a while. Opt for flavored tea such as peppermint, chamomile and lemon, sipping on which will be a soothing experience in itself.

- If you still feel like munching on something even after you've adequately hydrated yourself, go ahead and treat yourself with a lemonade slushy bowl. This is a trick that I learned from Sarah Tribett's YouTube channel and it has done wonders for me. It basically gives you something to chomp on without breaking your fast (Bonus points if you're a lemonade lover like me!).

Simply put some ice and a little water in a blender. Pour some fresh (or pre-packaged) lemon juice into it and a bit of stevia extract for sweetness. Now blend everything together and you have your very own lemonade slushy bowl to munch on. These slushy bowls are great because they make you think that you're eating something when its really just frozen lemonade that you're chewing on.

- Brush your teeth.

I know that you know; brushing is good for our oral hygiene. But how does it help with those food cravings that seem out of control by now?

The minty taste of your toothpaste can help curb food cravings. Not only can it distract your brain from craving sugar because mint has a slightly sweet taste to it, brushing your teeth after your last meal can also subconsciously make further eating undesirable. This is because we humans are lazy by nature and the thought of brushing our teeth again after another round of eating makes us think 'well, who wants those bagels anyway?!'

Brushing your teeth and cleaning your tongue also washes off any and all of the leftover taste from the food you last ate. It can therefore take your mind off from craving any more foodstuff.

- If all else fails, sleep it off. I know that you'll miss out on binge watching your favorite season if you go to bed now, but sometimes that is the only solution to help you avoid breaking your fast for the umpteenth time.

  Life isn't fair. And sometimes you have to make little sacrifices for the greater good.

Hack #6- Take baby steps and experiment

This is one of the most important hacks that you can use as a beginner or as someone who wants to transition into a different but advanced IF regimen (yet I don't know why it comes at #6).

When going for something that is more of a lifestyle change such as IF, you must give your body the time it needs to acclimatize itself to the new eating-fasting-eating situation. And there is a fairly easy way to do this. Just walk through the following steps that'll take you all the way from when you first start thinking about IF to a reasonably stable IF regimen that can be aced even as a beginner.

You can thank me later.

(Disclaimer: You might find that some of these steps were covered in earlier chapters. However, I have tried to break it all down into even smaller steps (hence called 'baby steps') to make it easier.)

- You must work on your mindset before anything else. Try to approach IF as a self-experiment in which you'll learn as you go. It's nothing that you must do to lead a healthy life, rather it's just another thing you're willing to learn about in your journey towards better health.

You may succeed or you may not. But that's okay because IF isn't for everyone. You can make your conclusions at the end of this exercise.

- Before you officially embark on the IF journey, you might want to pay a visit to your doctor to discuss any health conditions you have (or might have) in order to assess which version of IF is right for you.

- Remember, your first goal is to finish a fast. Take IF one fast at a time and to increase your chances of success, keep everything simple and easy. All the days and timings you've been hearing about are just for reference. Do what works best for you.

- Be prepared for making blunders. Most importantly, promise yourself that you'll let it go if you slip because slip-ups are normal.

- While you're still working on your mindset, decide on what you want to achieve with IF. This is extremely important because your goals will act as a lighthouse to guide your efforts regarding IF and help you measure the results you'll be achieving with IF.

Now that you've prepared yourself for what lies ahead, let's begin fasting intermittently. Remember, baby steps are all you must take, so here's how to do this:

1. For your first day, try to have a hearty dinner and don't eat anything after you have it. If you dine early (i.e. around 6 or 7 pm), you might be tempted to eat some snacks before bed. Curb your cravings by brushing your teeth as soon as you've eaten and have some flavored (but unsweetened) tea.

   Remind yourself that you're fine since you ate normally all day and even had a fulfilling dinner. There shouldn't be any reason to eat again.

2. Now that you're on your second day, aim to delay breakfast as long as you can.

   If you're wondering about what you've achieved on your first day of IF, it's this; by eating nothing after dinner and waking up at 7am the next day, you've already fasted for 12 hours straight! This might seem like a piece of cake because it really is. All you had to do was sleep through it and you're already fasting for half the day (i.e. 12 hours).

   As for when to grab your breakfast, try to have some water, coffee or tea until you find the time to relax and have your first meal of the day when the morning hubbub has died down a little. This may be 9 am or 10 am, whatever suits you.

Once you've successfully delayed your breakfast, you might find that you aren't craving lunch until 2 pm. That's perfectly fine. Listen to your body and act accordingly.

You've got this!

After you return home and sit down to eat dinner at 7pm, repeat what you did yesterday i.e. don't eat anything after dinner. And there you go, you're acing 14-15 hours fasts before you know it!

That wasn't so bad, was it?

3. Today is your third day of IF and your goal is to put an end to your snacking. You aren't eating after dinner and delaying your breakfast already. What you need to do now is to try and stop guzzling on snacks between lunch and dinner.

   This might seem daunting at first, but it really isn't.

   Come to think of it, we mostly snack because we don't have anything better to do or are simply sad and want to drown our worries in that pint of ice cream. Instead of listening to that little voice inside your head which says that you need to munch on something, try to remind yourself that you'll be having dinner in a few hours' time. Therefore, its unwise to blunt that hunger with some garbage snacks when a fulfilling dinner awaits you at home (remember meal-prepping? That comes in handy at times like these!).

More often than not, our bodies confuse thirst with hunger. Grab on some water or drink some unsweetened black tea and coffee to hydrate yourself and you might find that that hunger cue is gone.

Most importantly, try to keep yourself busy. Engage in some productive work or distract yourself with a phone call. This is one of the reasons it is recommended that you fast on weekdays so time flies by, and before you know it, its dinner time!

Don't forget to repeat what you've been doing for the past few days (no eating after dinner and a late breakfast) while adding on the no-snacking custom you've just set for yourself.

4. Today is day 4 of your IF regimen and you already feel a lot more confident than when you had just started.

   You're elated because you're doing almost 15 hours of fasting with no snacking in between and you feel like you've already come a long way.

   You've also realized a bunch of things at this point; mindful eating is completely possible, we often eat unnecessarily and out of habits or emotions and that hunger pangs go away if you don't entertain them.

   Now let's move on to the next step which is skipping breakfast.

I know. This one feels really scary.

You might ask, how can I function without breakfast, presumably the most important meal of the day? But you can.

Just push it through for one more hour and have lunch at, say, 11AM. Moreover, repeat everything you've built on this far; no eating after dinner, skip breakfast (this one is new!), have an early lunch instead of breakfast and don't snack between lunch and dinner.

At this point, you should be doing at least 16 hours of fasting.

Now that's some huge achievement!

5. After doing all of the above, step 5 just involves repeating everything you've learned and accomplished up until now and slowly letting your body acclimatize to this new eating pattern.

   Here's what a typical day in your life might look like at this stage:

   - Having dinner at 7 pm and eating nothing after that.
   - Pushing breakfast one hour later and having lunch at that time instead.
   - Eating nothing between lunch and dinner except drinking water, black coffee and tea (unsweetened).

- Eat, fast, eat. Rinse, repeat.

And there you go! You've successfully completed almost 16 hours of fasting daily. Don't underestimate yourself because this amounts to the same number of fasting hours as proposed by one of the most popular and user-friendly methods of IF i.e. 16:8 fasting.

If you still find that IF isn't for you, just give it a try for at least 3 more weeks after which you'll be free to choose whatever course of action suits you. I'd always encourage experimenting though. Sometimes the most mainstream and popular IF methods may not work for some and other IF methods will do the trick.

Hack #7- Use IF affirmations

You might have heard that anything can be achieved if you have the right mindset. And that is equally true for IF.

As we have discussed earlier as well, IF is a lifestyle change that puts your mind at work not only about when you're eating but also about what you're eating. It helps you make mindful decisions about the food you put in your body and see where this takes you.

But I'll be honest. This can be challenging.

Not only because fasting itself is a rather strenuous business (at least in the beginning) but also because we face countless temptations in our everyday lives that can make us think if we're putting ourselves through some undue hardship.

But knowing the virtues of IF, its hard to believe that the above is true.

How then do you battle the everyday temptations, wavering willpower and the deepest desires to indulge in all kinds of food available to you 24*7?

Through IF affirmations.

These affirmations are like that pep talk you give yourself before anything big in your life is about to happen or when you want to pull yourself together after feeling exceptionally down.

But for these to work, you must believe that they can. You must embody them with your own being and repeat them frequently enough to keep reminding yourself about them.

Only then can these break you free from temptations and bring about adamant behavior.

Sidenote: The affirmations below are just meant for inspiration. You can use them if they work for you or create your own that address the particular challenges you face in your life.

I want to lose weight and be healthy because I love myself

I want to live a healthy and long life

I am in control of my mind and body

My body is a sacred temple, the sanctity of which I'll respect

I deserve a healthy mind and body

I can resist temptation because I respect my body

Just as weight gain takes time, I know that weight loss will also take time, energy and commitment

The more I eat mindfully, the more I feel healthy and in control

Exercise and meditation is me time. I deserve it

I already have an amazing body. I just need to take care of it to maintain that

Eating healthy is a choice I deliberately make because I know it is good for me

If you look closely at the above affirmations, they'll seem like everything you would want to tell yourself every single day. And that's where the power of these affirmations lie. They allow you to inculcate ideal behavior and thoughts that you only wished you could have, except that now you're actively working towards making these a reality by repeating these affirmations to yourself every day or even multiple times a day.

If you feel like these sound a little silly, just go ahead and try them. With time, you'll start believing in these and most importantly, believing in yourself and your ability to change your life

For the better.

The Beginning

Yep.

This chapter heading isn't wrong or misplaced.

With the correct step by step approach and the correct mindset taken to intermittent fasting, it would not be too far of a stretch to say that your health would have taken on a brand new beginning.

Think of it like a reboot of sorts, or maybe a refresh perhaps.

Intermittent fasting brings on many great benefits, both tangible and intangible. For me, the start was the very obvious healthy weight loss, and the even better news was that the weight loss was of the sustainable sort. Not the lose it and rebound within three months kind!

Couple all that with increased mental alertness as well as better overall health, you can have loads to look forward to when you get plugged in well and proper into the intermittent fasting lifestyle!

But you have got to know something.

I may not have told you everything...

I have a confession to make before we end this book together.

I gave up on IF!

And it wasn't that I'll-try-it-some-other-day giving up.

I gave it up for good (and all) in the early stages of my IF journey.

IF had been challenging for me, like that one time when I wasn't able to lose weight even after three months of fasting intermittently (we've gone over this before) or those numerous instances of social encounters marked with consumption of calories (think birthdays, weddings and office celebrations) where apparently everything needs to be commemorated by eating/drinking something.

So this time, it was real. And I had decided that I wasn't coming back to the practice anytime soon.

Or maybe never.

You must be wondering what went so wrong so as to make me give up on IF altogether in that early period of time?

Honestly, the reasons were many.

First and foremost, I jumped into IF without knowing what to expect. And that's on me because I didn't do my homework. Secondly, I was breastfeeding my 6-month old at the time (I know, what was I even thinking?), juggling between two jobs and freelancing every now and then while crashing at a friend's place after leaving my parent's house out of extreme guilt (I was a 34-year-old with a newborn who couldn't make ends meet despite two jobs).

Fasting intermittently felt like I was torturing myself unnecessarily (obviously, I was doing it wrong!) and added to my already skyhigh pile of misery. Of course, had I known how to do it correctly (or NOT do it while breastfeeding an infant) and did my research more exhaustively, I could have saved myself the agony.

And the point of sharing this well-kept secret with you, as we wind this book up, is precisely this:

So you don't make the same mistakes that I did.

Such mistakes are costly in that they sometimes deviate you from things that might be actually good for you. *I know this because when I did it right,* IF reaped some amazing health benefits for me, both physically and mentally.

And it might very likely be that case for you as well.

So this book is meant as a guide to share what I've learnt in my IF journey and to (hopefully) save you from some of the headaches I got along the way.

IF is not for everyone and it should never be treated as a miracle cure for all the ills and diseases of the world. And i've said it a few times now.

But if you're someone who made a wrong move at the wrong time by jumping into the practice when they shouldn't have, then you'll only be disappointed. Whereas, if you do your due diligence and keep your head in the game, then you're all in for success.

And I hope that this book will help you achieve just that.

Cheers.

Made in the USA
Monee, IL
17 June 2021

71613531R00097